Coping with Aggressive Behaviour

Jane McGregor, PhD, is a freelance writer and a former university lecturer. In 2006, she was awarded a Wellcome Trust PhD studentship to study at the London School of Hygiene and Tropical Medicine's Centre for History in Public Health. She successfully completed her studies in 2010. Jane has published widely on the topic of addiction and addiction treatment and co-authored two self-help books, *The Empathy Trap: Understanding antisocial personalities* and *Coping with Difficult Families*, both published by Sheldon Press. She is a trustee of the Society for Research into Empathy, Cruelty and Sociopathy (SoRECS), a charity she is very passionate about.

Overcoming Common Problems Series

Selected titles

A full list of titles is available from Sheldon Press,
36 Causton Street, London SW1P 4ST and on our website at
www.sheldonpress.co.uk

101 Questions to Ask Your Doctor
Dr Tom Smith

Asperger Syndrome in Adults
Dr Ruth Searle

The Assertiveness Handbook
Mary Hartley

Assertiveness: Step by step
Dr Windy Dryden and Daniel Constantinou

Backache: What you need to know
Dr David Delvin

Birth Over 35
Sheila Kitzinger

Body Language: What you need to know
David Cohen

Bulimia, Binge-eating and their Treatment
Professor J. Hubert Lacey, Dr Bryony Bamford
and Amy Brown

The Cancer Survivor's Handbook
Dr Terry Priestman

The Chronic Pain Diet Book
Neville Shone

Cider Vinegar
Margaret Hills

Coeliac Disease: What you need to know
Alex Gazzola

Confidence Works
Gladeana McMahon

Coping Successfully with Pain
Neville Shone

Coping Successfully with Prostate Cancer
Dr Tom Smith

Coping Successfully with Psoriasis
Christine Craggs-Hinton

Coping Successfully with Ulcerative Colitis
Peter Cartwright

Coping Successfully with Varicose Veins
Christine Craggs-Hinton

Coping Successfully with Your Hiatus Hernia
Dr Tom Smith

Coping Successfully with Your Irritable Bowel
Rosemary Nicol

Coping When Your Child Has Cerebral Palsy
Jill Eckersley

Coping with Asthma in Adults
Mark Greener

Coping with Birth Trauma and Postnatal Depression
Lucy Jolin

Coping with Bowel Cancer
Dr Tom Smith

Coping with Bronchitis and Emphysema
Dr Tom Smith

Coping with Candida
Shirley Trickett

Coping with Chemotherapy
Dr Terry Priestman

Coping with Chronic Fatigue
Trudie Chalder

Coping with Coeliac Disease
Karen Brody

Coping with Diverticulitis
Peter Cartwright

Coping with Drug Problems in the Family
Lucy Jolin

Coping with Dyspraxia
Jill Eckersley

Coping with Early-onset Dementia
Jill Eckersley

Coping with Eating Disorders and Body Image
Christine Craggs-Hinton

Coping with Envy
Dr Windy Dryden

Coping with Epilepsy in Children and Young People
Susan Elliot-Wright

Coping with Gout
Christine Craggs-Hinton

Coping with Hay Fever
Christine Craggs-Hinton

Coping with Headaches and Migraine
Alison Frith

Coping with Heartburn and Reflux
Dr Tom Smith

Coping with Kidney Disease
Dr Tom Smith

Overcoming Common Problems Series

Overcoming Common Problems Series

Overcoming Common Problems

Coping with Aggressive Behaviour

DR JANE McGREGOR

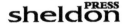
sheldon PRESS

First published in Great Britain in 2017

Sheldon Press
36 Causton Street
London SW1P 4ST
www.sheldonpress.co.uk

The author and publisher have made every effort to ensure that the
external website and email addresses included in this book are correct and
up to date at the time of going to press. The author and publisher are not
responsible for the content, quality or continuing accessibility of the sites.

British Library Cataloguing-in-Publication Data
A catalogue record for this book is available from the British Library

ISBN 978-1-84709-431-5
eBook ISBN 978-1-84709-432-2

Typeset by Fakenham Prepress Solutions, Fakenham, Norfolk NR21 8NN
First printed in Great Britain by Ashford Colour Press
Subsequently digitally reprinted in Great Britain

eBook by Fakenham Prepress Solutions, Fakenham, Norfolk NR21 8NN

Produced on paper from sustainable forests

Contents

Acknowledgements

My thanks go to psychiatrist Dr Marcia Sirota of the Ruthless Compassion Institute for sharing her ideas on dealing with aggression in everyday life. My thanks also go to Dr Claire Hardaker, lecturer in Forensic Corpus Linguistics at Lancaster University, who kindly shared her research on aggression in computer-mediated communication, specifically on trolling and cyberbullying. Last, but in no way least, thanks also to Fiona Marshall, my commissioning editor at Sheldon Press, for her steadfast support.

Introduction

Aggression is a complex issue, not least because what one person sees as an acceptable way to express anger or frustration may be seen by others as an aggressive act. So what is it that makes some people become so worked up over things that others would find fairly trivial?

All one has to do is check Twitter or some other social media. People seem to be so angry with their lot. On any day of the year, some individuals will have got very angry at someone for something they have said or written and sent them a nasty, threatening message. Other people then will become very angry at the individuals who sent the threats and at Twitter and social media in general for not doing more to stop it. A high-profile person intervenes and makes a protest about the way social media is being used by aggressors and this person's actions stimulate other people to write rage-fuelled messages challenging them. People then get back at the people who write rage-fuelled comments. The hostilities escalate, then abruptly cease and so it goes on, in relentless fashion. Is it harmless goings-on or is it toxic and something that needs to be curbed?

Some people rant over the slightest thing while others are slow to react. Some people sit on anger for a long time before they let rip, while others never seem to get angry and remain impassive. Is there a right way to do anger or get cross and express outrage? This book explores the different ways in which people express anger. A practical book, it shows you how to transform your approach to expressing and dealing with anger, especially if you most commonly are left dealing with aggression as opposed to anger. This includes your own aggression as well as other people's. The book considers commonly encountered forms of aggression: passive aggression, covert aggression, open aggression and outright hostility. It also discusses strategies for dealing with aggressors, as well as your own anger and frustrations in daily life.

Anger versus aggression

'Aggression' is not the same as 'anger', though people readily confuse the two. You can be very aggressive and mug someone in the street, but you needn't be angry with the person to perform this callous act. It is far more likely that the motivation behind this behaviour is wanting any valuables that person is carrying. Conversely, one can be angry with someone and not be aggressive towards them.

'Aggression' is often defined as any behaviour directed towards another individual that is carried out with the intent to cause harm. Perhaps someone is doing or saying something you don't like, so you do something to that person in a bid to stop them doing or saying it, such as threaten them with violence. That is aggression.

'Anger' is the state of emotional and physiological arousal. It can be experienced as an intense emotional response. It has been described as a feeling that involves a strong uncomfortable and emotional response to a perceived provocation.

Anger may have physical effects. It may increase our heart rate, blood pressure and levels of the hormones adrenaline and noradrenaline. Anger is thought to trigger part of the fight or flight brain response. The external expression of anger can be found in facial expressions, body language, physiological responses and, at times, acts of aggression. Psychologists view anger as a primary emotion experienced by humans and something that is necessary for survival. Anger can mobilize psychological resources to enable us to take action to help ourselves, but, on the less positive side, uncontrolled anger and acts of aggression can negatively affect personal or social well-being.

A brief history of anger

Around the year AD 180 Roman physician Claudius Galen (AD 130–210) made the following observations about anger:

> When I was still a young man . . . I watched a man eagerly trying to open a door. When things did not work out as he would like them, I saw him bite the key, kick the door, blaspheme, glare wildly like a madman and all but foam at the mouth like a wild boar. When I saw this I conceived such a hatred for anger that I was never thereafter seen behaving in such an unseemly manner because of it.[1]

Galen was not the first to note a dislike of uncontrolled anger. In around 350 BC, Aristotle also was troubled by unbridled anger, though he regarded anger as having a useful role when it arose as a result of injustice. He perceived it as a useful means of preventing wrongs, while he saw the opposite of anger – passivity – as insensitivity.[2] Emotions were regarded at this time as forms of appetite. Appetite was among the faculties or attributes that were collectively known as the common faculties, which included nutrition, sensation and locomotion. The uniquely human faculty was viewed as being the mind, involving reason and the will. It was thought that the mind could override appetite. This line of thought influenced later civilizations and thinkers. The general negative view of anger prevailed, even until the Middle Ages.

The writings of philosophers in ancient Greece suggest that uncontrolled anger was not uncommon in society, if the plays from those times are anything to go by. It is almost impossible to find an ancient Greek play or tragedy that doesn't involve a vicious murder or fury erupting in one of the characters. Yet anger was especially unloved by the Stoics. Stoicism is a school of philosophy that was founded in Athens in the early third century BC. Stoic doctrine was popular and had a following in Roman Greece and throughout the Roman Empire. The Stoics taught that destructive emotions such as anger resulted from errors in judgement and a person of moral and intellectual superiority would not suffer such emotions. Visual signs of anger were looked on with disdain. For example, red-faced or red-haired people were perceived as hot-tempered, which was said to be owing to hot and dry humours. The Stoics also regarded anger as worthless expenditure of effort, even in war or sport. It was considered a mistake and unwise to get angry. So harshly was uncontrolled anger regarded that suicide was considered preferable to raging!

In medieval times, the prevailing view was that restraint was a virtue. The idea was that as a mind was needed for people to get angry, the mind and will afforded humans control over their anger. This idea was taken up by Christians. A central idea of the Church was that humans had free will and were responsible for their behaviour and the consequences of it. This idea was picked up by Thomas Aquinas in his work *Summa Theologiae*, in which he described the habits of the mind that dispose people to evil or virtue.[3] Yet it was also acknowledged that people could find themselves overwhelmed by passion, including anger. In such instances, they were held to be insane and not responsible for their actions.

During the medieval period, it was popular to regard women and children as more prone than men to emotional displays. This was believed to be caused by a lack of moral education. Men were schooled in the idea that it was their responsibility to avoid getting angry. If someone provoked or slighted another, it was both individuals' responsibility to keep a sense of proportion and strive for balanced awareness by hearing the whole story. When dealing with other people's anger, the individual was advised to consider the situation from the angry person's perspective. Today, we might call this putting things into perspective and making use of our empathic abilities. Christians were encouraged to teach their children self-control. Humiliation was to be avoided, as was pampering and indulging children, especially boys. Training was done by the father, but other members of the household would join in, too. If a child was easily roused to anger, he would be punished for the loss of self-control.

There really hasn't been much of a shift in thinking since then. Expressions of anger towards those of higher status are still often prohibited as they may constitute a challenge to the social hierarchy. One of the social nuances children learn is that of deference and who might be considered an appropriate target for anger.

Periodically there are upsurges in anger in society. It makes people ask, 'What the world is coming to?', because it seems to spread in a socially contagious way. In recent history, for example, an escalation in aggression led to the Holocaust and, more recently, there have been terrorist attacks in many countries and places throughout the world.

Early twentieth-century Europe saw many angry days before, during and after the two world wars. For the political leaders of the period there was much to be gained from displaying anger and moral indignation. The then British Prime Minister, Winston Churchill, provided some fine examples of anger expressed for political purposes and expediency. In December 1914, warships entered British waters and fired hundreds of shells on Scarborough and several other coastal towns. Churchill expressed grief at first at the many lives lost, many of whom were children. Then later, in a letter to the Mayor of Scarborough, he branded the Germans 'the baby-killers of Scarborough'. A huge public outcry followed and the expression 'Remember Scarborough!' became a rallying call for allied troops in the First World War.

The Second World War, however, wasn't all about rousing anger and passions. A more stoic approach was evident in the wartime slogans, such as the popular poster 'Keep Calm and Carry On', produced by the British government in 1939 in preparation for the war. The poster was intended to raise the morale of the British public as the country was threatened with widely predicted mass air attacks on major cities.

In the immediate post-war period of the 1950s, there emerged a wave of 'angry young men'. The works of an assortment of playwrights and novelists, including John Osborne, who wrote the play *Look Back in Anger*, epitomize the era. These young writers had survived the Second World War only to find themselves in a struggle of a different kind in which their imagined future was being held back by outmoded social conventions. Anger at the older generation and demands for social change continued into the 1960s, when young people in the mainstream began to revolt against the norms of the time. The 1960s was also the decade of hippies and the anti-war movement, which was initially based on the older 1950s peace movement in the United States. In fact, the hippies were reviving and popularizing for a new generation the bohemian adventures of unconventional people of the preceding century. 'Peace' became synonymous with hippies; there was little place for anger in this subculture other than in the form of peaceful protest. The 'sit-in' and slogans such as, 'Make love not war' were synonymous with the movement.

Even in the late twentieth century, there was a tendency for anger to be viewed as a powerful emotion that was best avoided. In part this was because, from the 1980s on, anger was linked to antisocial behaviour. Writers published work highlighting the role of anger in hostilities of the period. Psychologist James R. Averill claimed that anger was antisocial, negative, unpleasant and very common.[4] It seemed to be a global problem, contagious and, for reasons unknown, it had reached crisis point. Quite often the problem appeared to be linked to economic and social issues. In the 1980s, daily life in the UK was set against a backdrop of riots, economic instability, high unemployment and social unrest. A negative reaction to anger and aggression was also evident in other countries.

An important cross-cultural study undertaken in the 1980s supported the idea of anger being commonplace and identified some key precursors. These included a breakdown in friendships, threats from strangers, unjust treatment, the violation of norms and damage to property.[5] As anger and aggressiveness emerged as dangerous elements, there was concern about children's exposure to aggressive behaviour in the media. Aggressive lyrics in popular music and the graphic violence of video and internet games common by the 1990s raised further concern about aggression and its pervasiveness in culture.

At the tail end of the century, there was renewed interest in the study of emotions. Emotion theorists – notably Richard Lazarus – theorized that anger was important in preserving self-esteem.[6] He suggested that before an emotion such as anger occurs, people make an automatic, often unconscious, assessment of what is happening and what it may mean for them and other people. From that perspective, anger becomes not just a rational but also an important component of survival. More recently still, anger increasingly has been linked to aggression via biology – in particular, neurobiology – but, in truth, many disciplines engage in the study of emotions. Human sciences study the role of emotions in mental processes, disorders and neural mechanisms. In psychiatry, emotions are examined to enable advances in the treatment of mental disorders. Emotions are studied to aid the approaches that might be taken and the provision of holistic health care. Psychologists examine emotions by treating them as mental processes and explore the underlying physiological and neurological processes. In neuroscience, scientists study the neural mechanisms of emotion by combining neuroscience with the psychological study of personality, emotion and mood. Linguists and educationalists also consider the role of emotions, in relation to learning and language. This is a fortunate happenstance as it provides an opportunity to draw on research findings from a wide range of disciplines in this book.

Anger in our times

What makes people angry in daily life? In all probability, as in times past, the primary culprits are other people. Some people rage like blast furnaces all the time, seemingly overreacting to what's going on around them. If your body can't distinguish between ordinary frustrations in daily life and truly life-threatening stress, it gears up to every challenge every single time. Our bodies get busy just in case we need to put up a fight or make a fast exit and release cortisol in readiness to do something physical.

Social convention of the day still has it that we should 'keep calm and carry on', even if that means paying no regard to our bodily reactions. The rise in popularity in the past decade of this slogan, originally printed on posters at the start of the Second World War, is an interesting phenomenon. Despite 2.5 million of the posters being printed, it was never displayed publicly; nearly all of them were pulped. Rediscovered in the aftermath of the financial crisis of 2007–2008, the words perhaps reflected something about British pluck and the will to turn economic downturn into recovery.

Subduing our emotional reactions and anger in a bid to keep calm and not look a fool by overreacting when there is no real trouble afoot is not without risk, however. We may be mindful of the need to calibrate our anger these days, but this has led to many of us feeling confused about when we can show anger. On the one hand, we might view anger as a mobilizing force for good (righteous anger or indignation). On the other hand, anger is often perceived as a strategy of manipulation to gain social influence and is regarded with deep suspicion. The end result is that anger is often viewed as problematical and a negative emotion. That is why many people fear losing control, going off the deep end and looking stupid.

This has led to people seeking ways to curb and manage their anger. Men, in particular, are encouraged to find non-violent ways of expressing their anger and anger management classes have become a favoured approach. Self-exploration of the situations that lead to anger is encouraged. Therapists issue advice on stress-reduction techniques and tips to acquire mindfulness (or, put another way, a state of conscious awareness), while assertiveness, which doesn't exactly equate to anger and aggression but relates to them, is encouraged in training programmes and self-help publications. Being essentially agreeable and pro-social has been promoted as good for health and well-being, yet researchers involved in a recent study published in the *Journal of Personality* discovered something surprising: those who are described as 'agreeable, conscientious personalities' are more likely to follow orders, including when instructed to deliver electric shocks that they believe can harm innocent people, than 'more contrarian, less agreeable personalities', who are more likely to refuse to hurt others.[7]

Without anger, it is hard to believe that we would be exercised or impassioned about much in life and it seems crucial for creativity. Volcanic rage is behind a lot of creative work. In a series of experiments published in the *Journal of Experimental Social Psychology*, it was demonstrated that anger promoted 'unstructured thinking' on a creativity task. A second experiment elicited anger directly in the subjects, before asking them to come up with ways to improve the condition of the natural environment. Once again, people who felt angry generated more ideas. Better still, their ideas were considered more original.[8]

Although in many situations people may feel uncivilized if they express uncontrolled anger, anger does have its purposes. It acts as a mobilizing force and can push us on towards accomplishing goals, even overcoming problems and barriers. In fact, when we see something as beneficial, we want it more when we are angry, or so a recent study by Dutch researchers suggests.[9] The expression of anger can also benefit and strengthen relationships. Pent-up and hidden anger has the reverse effect. That is because when anger is concealed, the other person in the relationship cannot know about it, so has less chance of doing anything to remedy the situation.

Anger also can help us develop insight. If we can notice when we get angry and why, this can motivate self-change. Anger is a strong social indicator that things are not right and need to be addressed. In this way, it can prevent violence. Good, righteous anger can lead to peaceful protest over out-and-out violence. Without the proper amount of anger, without moral indignation, we would lose the desire to protect our friends and our nation. Anger can also help us negotiate a better deal for ourselves and other people, but negotiating while also staying in control of our anger isn't easy. This has been a persistent problem for humanity; as the Greek philosopher Aristotle stated, 'Anybody can become angry – that is easy, but to be angry with the right person and to the right degree and at the right time and for the right purpose, and in the right way – that is not within everybody's power and is not easy.'

Anger and gender

Although men and women do not differ in experiencing anger, they do differ in their expression of it. Anger in men is often viewed as 'manly', especially when men act their anger out physically. Women usually get the message that anger is unfeminine and are encouraged to suppress it.

The notion that men express more anger than women is doubtful. In fact, research either supports the view that women express more anger than men do or reveals no gender differences.[10] Difference with respect to the expression of anger may largely be due to variation of social contexts. Different social contexts are likely to evoke different judgements about whether or not it is socially fitting to express anger, and it is likely that men and women differ with respect to the judgements they make. For instance, women differ from men in their perceptions of the social implications of expressing their anger.[11] One explanation for this is that men and women learn different rules for the expression of emotions. In general, girls are socialized to control hostile emotions and it seems that this is likely to lead them to hold off from displaying overt expressions of anger for fear of strong negative social criticism. Boys, by contrast, are socialized to express their anger freely.

What makes women angry most often are things that have common roots: powerlessness, injustice and the irresponsibility of other people.[12] It is not clear what factors trigger men's anger, but more is known about how they express it. Specifically, men tend to show physical aggression, passive aggression and impulsively deal with their anger. They also more often have a revenge motive for their anger. Women, however, tend to be angry for longer, can be more resentful and are less likely to express their anger than men. Women often use indirect aggression by not speaking to former friends and acquaintances again because of their anger.[13]

Outline of the rest of the book

There are implications for not changing our ways and not effectively dealing with our own and other people's hostilities; unfettered hostilities enacted on each other lead to social, emotional and health harms. Individually, we need to do our bit to scale it back and that is what this book is about.

What follows in the rest of the book? Chapter 1 takes a look at the experience of aggression and asks why anger is often expressed as aggression. Theories of aggression and the most commonly displayed forms of aggression are highlighted. The issue of online and cyber-aggression and the influences on online behaviour, including anonymity and other factors that interact with each other to create what is called the 'online disinhibition effect', are also discussed. By way of illustration, case examples are included.

Chapter 2 looks at the language of aggression and the verbal strategies aggressive people commonly employ, as well as non-verbal behaviour. Chapter 3 introduces ways in which to deal with hostility by making use of the language of empathy, as opposed to retaliating with aggression. There is some discussion of the empathy spectrum and how our default position on this spectrum affects our ability to see ourselves as other people see us and turn insight into action. There is an emphasis in this chapter on things we can do to improve our expression of emotions and our empathic abilities in order to lessen our aggression, become less self-absorbed and increase our sensitive awareness of and empathy for other people. Chapter 4 shows ways to respond to aggressors without aggression in online and everyday communication.

Chapter 5 addresses the common problem of passive aggression, while Chapter 6 looks at the insidious problem of covert aggression in online and everyday communication. Chapter 7 considers the more visible problem of overt aggression and hostility, again in online and everyday communication.

Chapter 8 gets us up to speed with the science of cruelty and discusses how to recover from relational and verbal forms of abuse and build emotional resilience. Finally, Chapter 9 looks at what's needed to help build a language of empathy in our culture.

Throughout the book dialogue taken from real life is provided, as well as practical solutions and ways forward. So let us now read on to Chapter 1, to look at why anger is so often expressed as aggression.

1

Recognizing aggression

Have you ever been struggling against a crowd of shoppers and got irritated because you need to reach the bus stop to catch the bus home? Other people won't allow you to pass by, so you end up barging into them. Someone gets shirty that you've pushed past them and the next thing you know, you are exchanging insults. The whole thing escalates, with others getting involved. This chapter is about situations like this – aggression in everyday life – and why it occurs so regularly.

Theories of human aggression

There are numerous theories behind human aggression. We share aspects of aggression with animals. Some people regard human aggression as deriving from a survival-seeking drive to stave off hunger or fear, as an aid to reproduction and as a means of gaining control over resources.

Genetics is not the sole cause of aggression, however. In recent years, increasing attention has been given to the way we are hard-wired. When we are in a reactive state, our brain signals the need for fight or flight. This means that we are unable to open ourselves to another person and even neutral comments may be taken as fighting words. Conversely, when we are in a receptive state, the brain sends messages to relax the muscles of the face and vocal cords, and normalizes blood pressure and heart rate. In this state, our social engagement system is switched on and helps us connect with others.

Not only regions of the brain but also chemicals in the brain have been linked with aggression, particularly neurotransmitters such as serotonin. Serotonin's role in impulsivity is well established. In addition, hormones are thought to play a role. Hormones are chemicals that circulate in the body and affect cells and the nervous system, including the brain. Testosterone is a hormone that is linked to the development of the male gender and physique and, in turn, has been linked to increased physical aggression, although its role is unclear. The general sway of research finds testosterone associated with behaviours or personality traits linked with criminality, but other studies on more general aggressive behaviour have found a relationship with testosterone in only about half the studies.

Less controversial is the involvement of the steroid hormones cortisone (a metabolite from cortisol, with a similar name, genesis and function) and testosterone in social aggression. The effects of these hormones seem to tap into aggressive approach (testosterone) and fearful withdrawal (cortisone), otherwise known as fight or flight. It is thought that the testosterone/cortisone ratio controls the balance between aggression and fear. In adults, reduced levels of cortisol are linked to lower levels of fear, or to a reduced stress response, which can be associated with more aggression. However, studies have found that in youngsters who exhibit aggression, some have abnormally high levels of cortisol, while others have abnormally low levels. So what is going on? It is thought that cortisol levels go up when individuals first become stressed or traumatized, but then decline again if they experience stress for an extended period. So it seems that the body adapts to long-term stress by blunting its normal response. In addition, the hormonal neuropeptides vasopressin and oxytocin – small protein-like molecules used by nerve cells to communicate with each other – may play a key role in complex social behaviours, including attachment and aggression. Vasopressin has been implicated in social aggression. Oxytocin may have a particular role in regulating female bonds with offspring and partners, including the use of protective aggression.

Aggression, though, varies from person to person and it is hard to explain in terms of what we know about the brain and as a result of scientific study alone. Similar groups of people with similar lived experience may, for instance, exhibit different patterns of aggression. With this in mind, and advancements in science and technology, there has been an increasing call for the integration of a range of scientific and social research to form a picture of the nature of human experience and reality.

Taking an historical perspective, what is striking is that, though aggression, conflict and violence sometimes occur, direct confrontation is generally avoided; humans find ways to socially manage conflict. Different rates of aggression or violence, currently or in the past, within or between groups, have been linked to the structuring of societies and environmental conditions, with influencing factors including the poor distribution of resources and population change.

One of the most enduring social theories of aggression is 'social learning theory', the originator of which was Albert Bandura. Bandura theorized that children learn aggression by observing the behaviour of others. There is a tendency for people to imitate the aggressive behaviour of others (sometimes called 'modelling'), especially where such behaviour is seen either to go unpunished or to be rewarded in some way. Social learning theory posits that when a favourable outcome, event or reward occurs after aggression, aggressive behaviour is strengthened.

From early infancy, children's aggression is typically expressed in temper tantrums and physical ways. In the general population, simple displays of direct aggression peak between two and three years of age and then decline, largely due to children's social and cognitive development. However, some children remain aggressive through adolescence and into adulthood. Aggressive adults may have poor social functioning and low pro-social behaviour. This leads some people to conclude that the development of aggression in childhood is socially learned.

Chief among theories in this area is 'coercion theory', which suggests that the development of aggression is largely explained by processes in which parents and children unintentionally train one another to be aggressive. Children are aggressive, parents demand compliance, children escalate their aggressive behaviour, then parents escalate their demands but yield to the child, tacitly reinforcing their children's aggressive behaviour.

'Social information processing theory' is another developmental model of aggression. This five-step model suggests that children encode and interpret cues. A highly aggressive youth may perceive his peers to be hostile. The steps include constructing a response, selecting a response and enacting that response; and that response is most often aggressive. This model has been further refined over the years.

Another theory of aggression is 'frustration-aggression theory', which suggests that when people are frustrated and cannot reach their goals, they become angry and behave in an aggressive manner. Environmental factors also play a role, including how people are raised. People who grow up frequently witnessing forms of aggression are more likely to believe that such violence and hostility are socially acceptable.

Social theories do not take into account potential biological factors influencing aggression, including genetics, biochemicals or neuroanatomical causes. It seems wise, then, to combine these theories to capture as many explanations of aggression as possible. The most comprehensive theory of aggression is the 'biopsychosocial model', which integrates biological, psychological and social perspectives. The model proposes that genetic bases and life experiences, possibly involving harsh treatment, rejection and failure, and family experiences that include poverty, instability and harsh discipline, converge to adversely affect an individual.

Aggression as a product of an anger system

At the root of aggression is an anger system. Anger is an essential human feeling and emotion. It is likely that we developed an anger system to protect and enforce our own interests against those of other people or creatures and threats from the environment around us. Ironically, if we did not have an anger system, in all likelihood we would not maintain our social networks or improve them. Anger allows us to express our concern about one another. In expressing our anger towards someone, that person may respond by apologizing or changing his or her behaviour, and that is how relationships can be repaired and improved. This happens at an individual level, in families and communities, and at national and international level, too. Anger may lead to war and conflict, but it also leads society to rectify or respond to social injustices.

Anger is activated by triggers and these triggers vary from person to person and by age, gender and culture. In women, anger is often triggered by their close relationships. For instance, they may feel let down by family members and friends. A man is more likely to be angered by objects that aren't working correctly, encounters with strangers and societal issues, according to studies conducted into anger and gender by Professor Sandra P. Thomas from the University of Tennessee.[1] Children's anger is most often roused when they are blocked from doing something they have set their minds on doing. We see this when children get worked up into a state of fury if their toys are taken away.

Anger, when it is emoted, encompasses everything from mild irritation to intense rage. When cartoon characters get angry, steam comes out of their ears. We say things such as, 'That makes my blood boil!' In real life, the response varies from individual to individual, but we may grind our teeth, clench our fists, go red and flushed. We may experience numbness or go pale, have tense muscles or get hot and clammy.

When we react to feelings of anger, chemicals such as adrenaline and noradrenaline surge through the body. In the brain, the amygdala (the part that deals with emotion) goes into overdrive. The time between a trigger event and a response from the amygdala can be a fraction of a second. Blood flow increases to the frontal lobe of the brain. This area controls reasoning and is likely to be what is keeping you from hurling objects across the room and smashing things. So this bodily reaction provides some balance and, more often than not, it prevents you from overreacting. If you are being activated constantly by triggers, however, then this state of alert can start to cause damage.

The nervous systems of the chronically angry are constantly working and can become overworked. Being chronically angry and hyper-aroused has health consequences. There is potential for liver and kidney damage, as well as high blood cholesterol levels. Anger may be accompanied by anxiety or depression, so such people are at greater risk of coronary artery disease and a heart attack.

Types of aggression

I have already mentioned several different types of aggression. Aggression, in general terms, is defined as harmful behaviour that violates social conventions and may include deliberate intent to harm or injure another person. I examine aggressive styles more fully in subsequent chapters, but here I provide descriptions of the sorts of aggression I refer to in the book. These types are overt, covert, verbal, passive and a newer form of aggression frequently displayed, online aggression, that can be overt or passive in form.

Overt aggression

Overt aggression involves outward or open confrontational acts of aggression, such as physical fighting, verbal threats and intimidation. Overt aggression consists of behaviours that are evident in early life and peak between the ages of two and three years. This aggression is derived from feeling intense anger and is sometimes called 'retaliatory aggression'. This form of aggression is not usually planned and often takes place in the heat of the moment. Say you are driving and another car cuts you up in traffic, if you begin yelling and berating the other driver, you are experiencing impulsive retaliatory aggression. Overt aggressive acts can include impulsive behaviours such as:

- hitting
- punching
- kicking
- biting
- pinching
- spitting
- hair-pulling
- pushing.

Physical injury to other people or self is not the only sort of harm or outcome of overt aggression. Overt aggression includes crimes to property, such as vandalism.

Overt aggression can also be 'instrumental aggression', sometimes called 'predatory aggression'. This is often carefully planned and exists as a means to an end. Hurting another person while doing a burglary is an example of this type of aggression. The aggressor's goal is to obtain money or acquire someone's possessions to sell on, and harming another individual is the means to achieve that aim.

Covert aggression

When a person is out to dominate or control, this may be done by using subtle or deceptive tactics to hide that person's true intentions. This is covert aggression, sometimes referred to as relational aggression. It can be a powerfully manipulative manoeuvre. Avoiding any overt display of aggression while simultaneously intimidating others into giving us what we want, it becomes a vehicle for interpersonal manipulation. Covert aggression is most often marked by surreptitious rule-breaking and antisocial acts, such as stealing, cheating and lying. Passive aggression and verbal aggression, as highlighted below, can be covert in nature. Covert aggression, in essence, is usually aggression performed in a clandestine way. For example, someone who is covertly aggressive may engage in private, one-on-one communication with the intended target, done in such a way that no one else overhears what is said. Other means may include the aggressor playing sadistic games as practical jokes or spreading malicious rumours. Covert aggression, including passive and verbal aggression, has received much less research attention than overt forms of aggression.

Verbal aggression

It seems that the school playground rhyme, 'Sticks and stones may break my bones, but words will never hurt me', may be wrong after all. Recent research by Martin Teicher from Harvard Medical School revealed that individuals who reported experiencing verbal abuse from their peers during childhood and adolescence had underdeveloped connections between the left and right sides of their brain, through the massive bundle of connecting fibres called the *corpus callosum*. This same group of individuals had higher levels of anxiety, depression, anger, hostility, dissociation and substance abuse than others in the study.[2]

Verbal aggression includes ridiculing, shouting at people, taunting, jeering, swearing and making threats. Some forms of verbal abuse, such as name-calling or sneering, are obvious; many more forms are covert, such as withholding or discounting, and much less easily detected as aggression. Verbal aggression may be carried out in a deliberately secretive way and often happens in private over significant periods of time. Prolonged verbal abuse can leave the targeted person very fearful and bewildered. Verbal aggression is usually part of a pattern that is difficult to recognize; we can be left with a feeling of confusion and upset without really understanding why. People who engage in verbal aggression use words (or silence) to gain and maintain control.

It is a form of aggression that is often not taken as seriously as other types because there is no discernible proof, and the verbal aggressor may effect a 'perfect' personality around other people.

In reality, however, verbal aggression can be more detrimental to a person's health than physical abuse. Examples include:

- spreading malicious gossip (direct, passive);
- refusing to speak (indirect, active);
- insulting others (direct, active).

Passive aggression

Passive aggression is characterized by passive resistance and an unwillingness to comply with expectations in interpersonal situations, at home or at work. It includes behaviours such as learned helplessness, procrastination, stubbornness, resentment, sullenness or repeated failure to accomplish requested tasks for which the individual is responsible. Examples of passive aggression include the following:

- refusing to speak or engage with others;
- refusing to perform a necessary task;
- acting as if you are incapable of helping yourself;
- saying you will do something, but coming up with endless excuses not to do it.

Online aggression

Online aggression is often seen when factors combine to change people's behaviour online. Six factors were described by psychologist John Suler in 2004 as the 'online disinhibition effect'.[3] These are:

- **dissociative anonymity** – 'My actions can't be attributed to my person';
- **invisibility** – 'Nobody can tell what I look like, or judge my tone';
- **asynchronicity** – 'My actions do not occur in real time';
- **solipsistic introjection** – 'I can't see these people, I have to guess at who they are and their intent';
- **dissociative imagination** – 'This is not the real world and these are not real people';
- **minimizing authority** – 'There are no authority figures here, so I can act freely'.

The combination of any number of these can lead to people behaving aggressively and in ways they perhaps would not if face to face.

Aggression in adults

Aggression in adults can be the result of many factors working together, but a number of conditions have been identified that can lead to the development of aggression. Among them are the ones described below.

Antisocial personality disorder (ASPD) ASPD is a personality disorder characterized by a long-standing pattern of disregard for and violation of the rights of others, and impulsive and aggressive acts. In the past, the terms 'sociopath' and 'psychopath' have been used diagnostically to describe individuals with this type of personality; nowadays neither of these terms is used as an official title of any diagnosis.

Individuals with ASPD or related disorders tend to have a pathological level of narcissism. Often their self-esteem is poorly regulated and they have a fragile and unstable sense of self. Emotion regulation is compromised by difficulties in experiencing, processing and moderating certain feelings, most especially anger, shame and envy. Relationships with other people are generally dysfunctional because they tend to protect and enhance their own self-esteem at the cost of cooperative relationships and intimacy. In consequence their actions are often determined by the dominance of aggression over shame. The disorder may be caused by a decreased sense of morals or conscience.

Narcissistic personality disorder (NPD) NPD is a personality disorder in which people are excessively preoccupied with personal adequacy, power, prestige and vanity, mentally unable to see the destructive damage they are causing to themselves and others. NPD was historically called megalomania and is a form of severe egocentrism. It is a disorder that is characterized by an overinflated sense of self-importance, as well as dramatic, emotional behaviour that is in the same category and style as in ASPD. Emotional outbursts and rage are often observed phenomena. Like those with ASPD, narcissists lack empathy. They are unable to relate to, understand and rationalize the feelings of others.

Everyday sadism This term is used to describe individuals who lack empathy and derive pleasure from watching or inflicting physical or psychological harm on others. This type of personality trait is more common than generally supposed, as many people have sadistic impulses, hence the term 'everyday sadism'. The type of personality is shown, for instance, in the colleague who repeatedly humiliates you and smiles while doing so, or who seems to reap pleasure from hurting you. Or it could be the person who plants seeds of discord on the internet (otherwise known as an internet troll) by starting arguments or upsetting people for fun. Researchers from the University of British Columbia recently conducted two online studies and found evidence that linked internet trolling with sadism.[4] A sadistic disposition is one that craves cruelty. Sadists find the act of hurting innocent people pleasurable and exciting, and they seek out opportunities to satisfy this appetite.

Borderline personality disorder (BPD) While not in the same league as the personalities in the 'dark tetrad' (the dark tetrad comprises the 'dark triad' of personality disorders – narcissism, psychopathy or sociopathy, Machiavellianism – together with sadism), and more for reasons of emotionally instability than sadistic bent, people with BPD are prone to lash out at others both verbally and physically during periods of anger and impulsiveness. Characteristics can include overwhelming feelings of distress, anxiety, worthlessness or anger; difficulty managing such feelings without self-harming, for example by abusing drugs and alcohol or taking overdoses; difficulty maintaining stable and close relationships; sometimes having periods of loss of contact with reality; and, in some cases, threats of harm to others.

Bipolar disorder People who have bipolar disorder may act aggressively during a manic phase. Additionally, while struggling with depressive cycles, people who have bipolar disorder may become highly irritable, leading to outbursts of aggression.

Schizophrenia While most individuals who have schizophrenia are not violent, occasionally the breaks in reality that characterize this disorder can lead to full-blown psychosis. During psychotic episodes, an individual may respond to internal stimuli and act aggressively towards others out of fear.

Substance use People with a prior history of violent behaviour may seek drugs in order to get stimulation and sustain an addiction.

However, those addicted to substances may experience bouts of aggression during intoxication. Stimulant drugs such as amphetamines can cause aggression during the high, which can be quite dangerous for the individuals and others around them. In addition, depressants such as alcohol and even prescribed antidepressants can cause aggressiveness, agitation, hostility, impulsivity and irritability.

Aggression can also occur when individuals are recovering from types of addiction. For instance, people who stop using tobacco products often feel agitated and may exhibit a short temper, impatience, and other manifestations of aggressive behaviour as the body goes through withdrawal.

Neurological conditions and brain injury Injuries to the brain can lead to the development of aggression. Severe trauma to the head causes the brain to bounce within the skull, which may lead to bruising that affects the brain's production of different types of neurotransmitters. Individuals may find they become overcome with intense feelings of anger, which is likely to cause them to lash out. Often, the behaviour diminishes as the brain heals, especially if medication is taken to help compensate for the imbalance of neurotransmitters.

Aggressive behaviour can also stem from the presence of some type of disease or brain disorder. People with autism may exhibit aggressive behaviour occasionally. In a similar way, people with epilepsy may become aggressive during certain phases of a seizure. In individuals with attention deficit hyperactivity disorder (ADHD), aggressive behaviour may develop out of sheer frustration.

Emotional trauma Emotional trauma can lead to fits of anger and rage. Following a traumatic event, individuals can experience an emotional imbalance that is partly manifested by bouts of aggressive behaviour. Therapy, along with medication, can often help move the healing process along, and aid recovery from the trauma. As the healing progresses, the episodes are likely to occur less frequently, along with becoming shorter and less intense. Seeking help sooner rather than later helps to minimize the damage that aggressive behaviour can do, especially in the area of personal relationships.

Aggression in older adults

Elderly people often face a multitude of medical and emotional problems, which can lead to the development of aggression. Those who are struggling with aggressive behaviours may have an underlying condition that causes them to act aggressively, such as Alzheimer's disease or psychosis.

Alzheimer's disease and dementia Dementia is not a single syndrome but a group of syndromes. Alzheimer's disease is the most common form of dementia in the elderly. It directly impacts the brain by destroying areas that are involved in emotional regulation. Thus, many who struggle with Alzheimer's disease engage in aggression and violence in the later stages of the disease – behaviour that is very often quite out of character. Individuals may be disorientated and not know where they are, lashing out at loved ones and caregivers, or become aggressive as a result of fear stemming from confusion.

Psychosis 'Psychosis' is a general term that refers to an altered mental state, including a break from reality. The elderly may experience this symptom as a result of existing medical conditions, medication interactions, or mental illness. The hallucinations and/or delusions characteristic of this mental state may cause an adult to lash out at others. Older adults who have psychosis frequently become violent towards themselves or others.

Case studies

As previously highlighted, some forms of aggression are direct and obvious, while other forms are more veiled. Below are examples of different sorts of aggression seen in everyday life.

Overt aggression

Case 1

Simon, 33, was jailed for two years after he attacked a neighbour. The incident happened as his neighbour was outside trying to repair his car. Suddenly Simon appeared on the scene in an angry and agitated state, having misplaced the keys to his flat. He had been seen repeatedly kicking his front door and shouting and swearing. His neighbour heard the commotion and asked him to calm down, as there were children in the vicinity, but he became aggressive towards his neighbour. He kicked his neighbour's car. Then he punched his neighbour in the face and knocked him unconscious. There were fears his neighbour might lose the sight in one eye.

Case 2
A cyclist shouts out in alarm as a car narrows the space through which the cyclist can safely proceed. The driver swears out of the window at the cyclist. Eventually the cyclist comes to a halt, as does the driver. The driver storms out of the vehicle and starts shouting at the cyclist. The driver loses his temper and accuses the cyclist of deliberately scratching the side of his car. At this point, the driver begins to mimic the cyclist and threatens to kill him. 'Did you f***ing scratch my car? I'll f***ing kill you. I'll f***ing smash your teeth. If people weren't watching over there [bystanders had begun to stop and stare on the other side of the road] I'd break your f***ing neck.'

Passive aggression

Steve is a very passive, restrained person who avoids confrontation at all costs. He is not good at asserting his opinion or expressing a view and hates small talk. He is pleasant to a fault. He doesn't ever admit to feeling angry about things, even if he has just cause to be angry or annoyed. Instead he just shrugs things off and trudges on. He has been this way for most of his life and, in recent years, his passivity has become his defining characteristic. He rarely has anything to say to anyone. He walks around with his shoulders hunched and his eyes cast down, which gives him the air of someone hard done by.

If asked, he would most likely describe himself as a supportive partner, but his wife of 18 years, Anne, doesn't find him so. She realizes, looking back, that she is the one who has made all the important decisions in their life together. He is unwilling to initiate anything, whether it is a big thing such as moving house, or a minor thing such as helping around the house or engaging with their two teenagers. He rarely initiates sex and makes her feel demanding, bothersome and needy if she seeks affection from him.

Anne finds she is increasingly annoyed and frustrated with his passivity. When she expresses her concern about their marriage and how unsupported she feels, Steve fails to comprehend what the problem is. He seems unconcerned about whether they stay together or go their separate ways. This leaves Anne feeling extremely frustrated.

All any discussion on the state of their marriage does is cause him to become moodier and more sullen. He has withdrawn any support around the house, even refusing to walk the family dog, and he frequently goes off sick from work. He speaks only when absolutely necessary and most of the time gives Anne the silent treatment. He's become quite the recluse and this leaves Anne in a quandary. She spends more and more time with her own social circle and recently confided in her friends that she is seriously considering leaving him.

Covert aggression

Mary, 84, has dementia. She lived in a care home and her family visited when they could. During one visit her daughter became concerned about bruises on her body and saw that she was more distressed than usual. When asked about the bruising, Mary complained that she had been slapped by the nurse on duty. The family were so concerned that they decided to install a covert camera.

Abuse spanning five days was captured on the hidden camera. It showed the nurse shaking Mary and verbally abusing her on a number of occasions. The video footage showed the nurse swearing at Mary and calling her a 'horrible old lady' and a 'nasty old cow'. It also revealed that the nurse had not given the pensioner her medicine properly, showed her striking Mary and shaking her before telling her to 'p*** off'.

At one point, along with an older female colleague, the nurse dragged Mary across her bedroom floor between her chair and bed, making the elderly woman scream in pain. The nurse threatened her with violence, then afterwards carried on chatting to her colleague. Mary was shrieking and visibly distressed.

Luckily for Mary, her ordeal soon came to an end. Her family reported the abuses on the footage to the authorities and both nurses were arrested and charged. One pleaded guilty to four counts of wrongly administering medicine, and both pleaded guilty to ill treatment by moving a patient in an unapproved manner. The two nurses subsequently were banned from ever again working with vulnerable adults.

Online aggression

In a real-life, high-profile case, a man retweeted menacing posts threatening to rape the MP Stella Creasy. This came after the MP campaigned to put the nineteenth-century novelist Jane Austen on the new £10 note.

The man used a number of Twitter accounts to retweet sinister posts and send a series of menacing messages directly to the MP. One message posted by him described the 'best way to rape a witch'. He also wrote: 'If you can't threaten to rape a celebrity, what is the point in having them?'

According to victim impact statements that were read out in court, Ms Creasy stated that she had been terrified about the threats. The prosecutor said that the man's messages had a substantial effect on Ms Creasy, who felt 'increasing concern that individuals were seeking not only to cause her distress but also to cause her real harm which led her to fear for her own safety'. The court heard that the MP had installed a panic button in her home following the incident.

Fortunately the online aggressor was found guilty of sending indecent, obscene or menacing messages and he was placed on a restraining order banning him from any contact with Ms Creasy. According to those who were present in court, the man showed no emotion as the sentence was passed.

Everyday sadism

Case 1: In daily life

Simon is a gay man in his early forties. For the past five years he has worked in a finance department, where he gets on well with his colleagues. However, about a year ago a new manager was brought in to run the department. This manager often undermines Simon and criticizes his performance. When no one else is in earshot he mutters nasty comments about his sexuality and one time he called him a faggot.

Simon has made numerous complaints about this man's conduct, but his complaints fall on deaf ears. Recently the harassment reached new heights when the manager told him, 'Everything was OK until you started working here in this department'. When Simon left work that day he found his car had been keyed and someone had written into the dust on the rear and boot of the car, 'No shirt-lifters here'.

Case 2: Online

In a real-life case of everyday sadism online, a 25-year-old man, an internet 'troll', caused untold distress by leaving obscene messages and videos on a condolence page set up by the family of a 15-year-old girl who had committed suicide.[5] He also hijacked tribute websites of three other children he had never met. Sadly, the traumas didn't stop there; one of his victims was wrongly accused by others of posting the messages and attempted suicide.

This was one of the first cases of its kind in the UK. The man admitted that he was hooked on the sick craze of 'trolling' – where internet users deliberately leave abusive and bullying comments on networking sites – and was sentenced to 18 weeks in prison and banned from using social networking sites for five years. Thankfully the teenager who had attempted suicide survived.

In the next chapter I look at different ways in which people act out their aggression and how to be more alert to aggressors in everyday life, whether in real life or online.

2

Common lines of attack

This chapter is intended to help you recognize the language of aggression and conflict. I hope that understanding what you are dealing with will give you a chance to deal with aggression in ways that don't leave you battle-scarred. First, let us take a look at the kind of personalities who most frequently engage in acts of overt and covert aggression.

Aggressors rely on the passivity of others

At times in life we may find ourselves lacking interest in or concern for other people or even ourselves. Some of us reach a point where we are emotionally unable to connect with ourselves and others. This is sometimes referred to as 'emotional numbing'. It can be a way and means of dealing with anxiety by avoiding certain situations that trigger it (psychologists sometimes call this 'dissociation' or 'depersonalization'). It can also be a decision to avoid engaging emotionally, typically for personal, social or other reasons.

A lack of responsiveness to our own or other people's safety can also occur because some individuals have difficulty identifying and describing emotions in themselves. They may experience difficulty both in identifying feelings and in distinguishing between feelings. Furthermore, they may have difficulty describing feelings to other people and/or have constricted ability to use their imagination or they may be externally orientated. This may be as a result of being unaware of what's going on inside themselves (lack of inner self-talk, an inability to reflect on their feelings and conduct, which in turn hinders self-awareness). Typically, individuals like this have a cognitive style of thought process and reasoning.

This lack of interest in others seems to go hand in hand with a culture of self-obsession. Being self-absorbed means that we can become blind, indifferent and apathetic to the people around us. The word 'apathy' is derived from the Latin *apathīa* (freedom from passion or feeling) and Greek *apátheia* (ἀπάθεια: from 'a-', without, and 'pathos', suffering or passion). Often it is a temporary affliction, as a first reaction to danger, for example. Apathy can be an avoidance strategy employed in the hope that the problem will go away. Or it can be the case that we ignore other people who are suffering because at that moment we don't view them as our equals. We view them instead as 'others', objects and 'its'.

Some argue that we live in an increasingly self-focused and narcissistic culture. Ours is a culture of 'me, myself and I', with less room for 'us and we'. The internet is 'I-centric' and gadgets and 'apps' reflect the rise of the 'I' culture and narcissism of our times: iTunes, iPod, iPhone and iPad.

All of us can be selfish at times, but some people are so self-preoccupied that they are unable to form healthy relationships. Being self-preoccupied is very common in adolescents, but most individuals grow out of this over time. Interestingly, and perhaps indicating how much behaviour is socially learned and influenced, a recent study carried out in Atlanta, Georgia, found that children who enter adulthood during recessions are 'less self-obsessed'. The study found that growing up during bad times 'dampens narcissism and entitlement'.[1]

It is tempting to look at self-absorption and apathy in relation to the lives of other people merely as a problem of the individual, but it is not. It is a problem of global proportions and extremely hazardous. This was demonstrated effectively in experiments of the 1960s when Stanley Milgram, a professor at Yale University, set out to test the human propensity to obey orders. In the experiment, a participant in the role of 'teacher' was asked to administer electric shocks, of increasing strength, to a 'learner' whenever the learner answered a question incorrectly. (The 'teacher' had been given an electric shock from the electro-shock generator as a sample of the shock that the 'learner' would supposedly receive during the experiment.) The experiment was stopped after the subject supposedly had been given the maximum 450-volt shock three times in succession (in fact, the learners did not receive a shock and were faking their physical response). In the experiments, 65 per cent of the 'teachers' administered the experiment's final massive 450-volt shock, though many were uncomfortable doing so. Milgram's experiments have been repeated many times over the years and yielded consistent results: a person of authority can strongly influence other people's behaviour, with appalling consequences. What we can take from this is that apathy can damage people and political systems. If, alternatively, we focus on others, our world expands.

Apathy and indifference can enable aggression and violence to occur in a culture and we can deterred from helping one another out. Milgram's obedience experiments indicate that two-thirds of us would potentially commit acts of violence or aggression based on the orders of a person of authority. This is a disturbingly high level of compliance. This propensity was shown to appalling effect in the 2012 docudrama *Compliance*, which was based on true events. A prank caller poses as a police officer and convinces the manager of a fast-food restaurant that one of her employees has committed a crime, and gets her to carry out intrusive and unlawful procedures on the employee. What *Compliance* shows is that when obedience and badly suppressed fear become the prevailing conditions and state of affairs, submitting is all too easy. At any time, and in any period, when people supposedly in authority tell us what to do – we do it.

It isn't just a propensity to follow orders that influences our passivity in the face and presence of violence and aggression. Another factor at play is the bystander effect.

The bystander effect

The bystander effect is sometimes referred to as bystander apathy and is a social psychological phenomenon that sees individuals not offer any means of help to a victim when other people are present. The greater the number of bystanders, the less likely it is that any one of them will help. Researchers have studied the phenomenon and attribute the occurrence of passive bystanding to a 'diffusion of responsibility': when people believe that there are other witnesses to an emergency, they feel less personal responsibility to intervene. They assume someone else will help. The end result is altruistic inertia. Researchers also suggest that we don't act on occasion due to the effects of 'confusion of responsibility', where bystanders fail to help someone in distress because they don't want to be mistaken for the cause of that distress. What's more, sometimes bystanders don't intervene in an emergency because they are misled by the reactions of the people around them. We succumb to what is known as 'pluralistic ignorance' – the tendency to mistake one another's calm demeanour as a sign that no emergency is actually taking place. There are strong social norms that reinforce this – the 'keep calm and carry on' mentality is one such. We adhere to these norms, because it's embarrassing to get in a panic when no danger really exists!

What can further compound the issue of whether or not we will help another person out is how comfortable we are about certain feelings in ourselves. Some people are fantastically empathetic and helpful when it comes to showing care and compassion for other people, but have very little empathy when it comes to dealing with someone's outrage. Some close down in the face of violence and abuse; some cut off completely from emotions they are frightened of in themselves. While passivity can be simply the first reaction to perceived danger and an avoidance strategy employed in the hope that the problem will go away, it can also be something more sinister, for example when people passively or actively connive in hostilities they witness. There are many reasons why people join forces with aggressors: they may fear punishment if they don't go along with the scheme; they themselves may bear a grudge towards the targeted person or persons; or they just feel no real connection with them and shut off from feeling concern because of this. Sadder still, they may go along with the situation on account of boredom or to revel in a sense of Schadenfreude! In such cases, apathy becomes not just a lack of empathy but also a betrayal of it.

Just-world effect

The 'just-world effect', sometimes called the 'just-world phenomenon', refers to people's tendency to believe that the world is just and people get what they deserve. Because people want to believe that the world is fair, they will look for ways to explain away injustice, often blaming the victim. Those with this belief tend to think that when bad things happen to people, it is because these individuals have done something bad to deserve their misfortune. Conversely, this belief also leads people to think that when good things happen to people it is because those individuals are good and deserve their good fortune.

There are reasons why people cling to the notion of a just world; the most obvious is that we don't like to think about ourselves ever becoming the victim of violent crime. Thus blaming the victims and viewing their actions and behaviour as somehow causing or justifying violence – say in cases of assault or rape – means that we can go on believing that we will never be the victim of such a crime ourselves, because we can simply avoid the behaviours of the victims, which caused harm to come their way. Another possible explanation is that people want to reduce the anxiety that is evoked by acknowledging injustices in the world. Believing that individuals are completely responsible for their misfortunes means that other people are able to go on believing that the world is just and fair.

Personalities low in empathy

All of us can be placed along the line of the empathy spectrum. In his book *Zero Degrees of Empathy*, Simon Baron-Cohen proposed that we imagine we each have an empathy circuit in the brain that determines how much empathy we have.[2] He also proposed that there is a spectrum of difference where empathic abilities go, and each of us is positioned somewhere along it. Baron-Cohen's research indicates that the majority of people have a default position where empathy and empathic abilities go somewhere in the middle of the spectrum (points 3 to 5, the spectrum ranging from 1 to 6, shown in Table 1). Some people lack empathy to such an extreme that they don't have concern for other people at all (personalities positioned at point 0). At the other end of the spectrum, some individuals possess an almost unstoppable drive to empathize (point 6).

Table 1 The points on the empathy spectrum

Point 0	No empathy and hurting others means nothing to them
Point 1	Capable of hurting other people but feels some regret if they do so
Point 2	Has enough empathy to inhibit them from acts of physical aggression
Point 3	Compensates for lack of empathy by covering it up
Point 4	Low to average empathy
Point 5	Slightly higher than average empathy
Point 6	Very focused on the feelings of others. An almost unstoppable drive to empathize.

Personality types that use aggression

The following personality types use aggression in their everyday interactions more frequently than the rest of us.

Everyday sadists

There are several personality types that are more likely to harm others than the average person would. Psychologists previously have talked about the 'dark triad' in personality, representing a combination of narcissism, psychopathy and Machiavellianism, the latter characterized by a duplicitous way of interacting, a disregard for morality and a focus on self-interest and personal gain. Now researchers are beginning to believe that, additionally, there is a kind of sadism that shows up in a more benign, commonplace form – everyday sadism.

A study carried out in 2013 at the University of British Columbia investigated the idea that everyday sadists are willing to inflict harm.[3] The researchers reasoned that people high in this less overt form of sadism might themselves become more aggressive when provoked than other individuals. To test their theory, they offered study participants a choice of several unpleasant tasks: killing bugs, helping the experimenter kill bugs, cleaning dirty toilets, or enduring pain from ice water. The bug-killing wasn't real, of course, though it was made to appear so for the experiment. Those with sadistic personalities were identified as the most likely to select the task involving killing, and they derived greater pleasure from the act than those who killed fewer bugs. Other studies have shown that those high in sadism are willing to be aggressive towards an innocent person when aggression is easy. What was disturbing is that out of all the personalities, only sadists increase the intensity of their attack once they realize people will not fight back.[4]

Examples of everyday sadism include:

- seeking to ruin another person's relationship or jeopardize someone's job;
- portraying someone in a false light in an effort to damage his or her reputation;
- intentionally excluding an individual from the 'in-group', such as a colleague or family member;
- bullying, including cyberbullying.

Stalkers

Stalking is a covert aggressive act. It is unwanted or obsessive attention by an individual or group towards another person. Stalking behaviours are related to harassment and intimidation and may include following victims in person or monitoring them. Stalking is illegal in many countries, but some of the actions that can contribute to stalking are not illegal in themselves, such as gathering information, calling someone on the phone, sending gifts, emailing or text messaging. They become illegal when they breach the legal definition of harassment. In the UK, the law states that incidents defined as harassment, when the stalker should be aware that their behaviour is unacceptable, only have to happen twice for it to be classed as illegal. Stalkers may use threats and violence to frighten their victims, engage in vandalism and property damage, or make physical attacks that are usually meant to frighten. The majority of stalkers are former partners. A Home Office research study found that the Protection from Harassment Act is mostly used to deal with a variety of behaviours relating to domestic and inter-neighbour disputes.[5]

A stalker's pursuit of victims can be influenced by various psychological factors, including anger, hostility and projection of blame, obsession, minimization, denial and jealousy. Conversely, it is commonly the case that the stalker has no antipathy towards the victim, but simply a longing that cannot be fulfilled due to deficiencies in their personality. According to a UK study, in 5 per cent of cases there is more than one stalker, while 40 per cent of the victims who participated said that friends or family of their stalker had also been involved. In 15 per cent of cases, the victim was unaware of any reason for the harassment.[6]

'Harassment' was criminalized in England and Wales by the enactment of the Protection from Harassment Act 1997. It makes it a criminal offence to pursue a course of conduct that amounts to harassment of another person on two or more occasions. The court can issue a restraining order, which carries a punishment of imprisonment if breached. In 2012, the government stated an intention to make another attempt to create a law aimed specifically at stalking behaviour, but as yet there are no changes to existing laws.

In Scotland, behaviour commonly described as stalking was prosecuted as the Common Law offence of breach of the peace before the introduction of the statutory offence against section 39 of the Criminal Justice and Licensing (Scotland) Act 2010. Either course can be taken depending on the circumstances of the case.

Cyberstalking is, as its name suggests, the use of computers or other electronic technology to facilitate stalking.

Individuals with antisocial personalities and narcissistic traits

Some people have little or no conscience or ability to empathize with the feelings of others. Terms used to describe absence of empathy or conscience (the moral-emotion apparatus most of us use to keep our conduct in check) include sociopath, psychopath, narcissistic personality disorder (NPD, where people have an inflated sense of self-importance and an extreme preoccupation with themselves) and antisocial personality disorder (ASPD). The medical profession continues to define and redefine the features of these conditions, but however these individuals' personalities and behaviours are defined, sharing your life with or becoming involved in some way with a person with one of these disorders can prove very traumatic and destructive.

It is understood that those personalities with definably antisocial traits have no qualms about hurting others, but they are more likely to do so when it serves a specific purpose. Individuals with narcissistic personalities and tendencies, and those who are wholly self-centred, grandiose and exploitative, also lack empathy. Not only are they excessively preoccupied with themselves, they often believe that they are unique or 'special'. They lure you in with their charisma and charm but, after sweeping you off your feet, they have no qualms in putting themselves first or in exploiting you for personal gain. Beneath the superior façade they can be fragile and unable to handle criticism. They compensate for this by belittling others or being cruel in order to validate their own self-worth. This said, narcissists, unlike everyday sadists and those with traits along the lines of ASPD, are less likely to be aggressive towards another unless their ego is threatened. Then they can implode with rage like you have never seen. Narcissistic rage is a sight one definitely does not want to behold!

Strategies used by aggressors in everyday life

Next I consider the ruses, specifically the verbal and non-verbal strategies, commonly employed by aggressive people to harass and maim their victims, beginning with gaslighting. Then, highlighted are some strategies most likely to be used by the individuals discussed in the case study examples from Chapter 1, including projection, denial, displacement, overt, passive and covert aggression.

Gaslighting

It is fairly common for people who are especially disagreeable and antisocial to use what are called 'gaslighting' tactics. Gaslighting is the systematic attempt by one person to erode another's reality. The syndrome gets its name from the 1938 British stage play *Gas Light* by Patrick Hamilton, also made into a film in 1940 and 1944. It features a murderer who attempts to make his wife doubt her sanity, using a variety of tricks to convince her that she is crazy so she won't be believed when she reports the strange things that are genuinely occurring. This includes, in particular, the dimming of the gas lamps in the house (which happens when her husband turns on the normally unused gas lamps in the attic to conduct clandestine activities there). The term has since found its way into clinical and research literature.

Gaslighting is a form of psychological abuse in which false information is presented in such a way as to make the target doubt their own memory and perception. It is a deliberate ploy that occurs between the two individuals – the covert aggressor and the target. The endgame is that the person being gaslighted thinks he or she is going crazy. Anyone can become the victim of another person's gaslighting moves. Gaslighting can take place in any kind of relationship – between parent and child, between siblings or friends or between groups of people including work colleagues. The process of gaslighting distorts our sense of reality and makes us disbelieve what we see.

Gaslighting may simply involve the denial by an abuser that previous abusive incidents ever occurred, or it could be the staging of strange events intended to disorient the target. In order to gain control and manipulate another person a covert aggressor will employ positive reinforcement tactics such as praise, approval, even sympathy to draw you in. Then the aggressor will create a growing climate of fear and self-doubt with the use of intermittent positive and negative reinforcement (threats, intimidation, even playing the victim) to disorient the targeted person. These are the tactics used to 'gaslight' another person. To be 'gaslighted' is to be left in a state of extreme bewilderment and anxiety.

The effect of gaslighting is to arouse such an extreme sense of anxiety and confusion in the targets that they reach the point where they no longer trust their own judgement. The techniques are similar to those used in brainwashing, interrogation and torture – the instruments of psychological warfare. This is Machiavellian behaviour of the worst kind. Targets exposed to it for long enough lose their sense of self. They may find themselves second-guessing their memory, becoming depressed and withdrawn and totally dependent on the abuser for any sense of reality. The process of gas-lighting distorts our sense of reality and makes us disbelieve what we see. Even when victims are bewildered, they are reluctant to see the gaslighter for what he or she is. Being blind to the reality of the true situation is essential for gaslighting to work. Gaslighting does not happen all at once; if you suspect you are in the early stages of being gaslighted by someone, you can protect yourself by walking away.

Projection

Accusing others of faults and shortcomings, while disowning one's own failings, is an example of projection. It is a common tendency to defend ourselves against unpleasant impulses by denying their existence in us while attributing them to others. For example, a person who is rude may constantly accuse other people of being rude. There is disregard for the other person or for how the pro-jected statements, true or false, affect that person. Here are some examples.

- **Blaming the victim** regarding a crime or incident as the fault of the victim for having attracted the other person's hostility.
- **Projection of guilt** a form of defence that may be linked to the making of false accusations. At the level of interpersonal rela-tionships, projection of guilt or a severe conscience is most often seen in cases of infidelity. The guilty partner may unconsciously

project on to the partner and accuse him or her of infidelity, in a process linked to denial.

- **Domineering behaviour and aggression** projecting one's own feelings of vulnerability on to other people. The aggressor's own sense of personal insecurity and/or vulnerability become aggressive projections of displaced negative emotions.

Scenario 1
Sally feels insecure about the outfit she has chosen to wear for a special occasion night out. It has cost her a lot of money, which adds to her distress about it. As she comes downstairs, she blurts out to John, her husband, 'Why are you looking at me like that? Don't you like this outfit?' His puzzlement is met with hostility and an argument ensues. Sally spends the rest of the evening sulking and blames John for ruining their night out. In this example Sally 'projects' her feelings onto her husband.

Scenario 2
You make a mistake at work that no one notices, but you feel so insecure about it that unwittingly you accuse a colleague of saying that you're incompetent and not up to the job. This causes a rift in the office and upset among your colleagues. Most people think you were needlessly hostile. Meanwhile you're left upset and feeling victimized. In reality no one has actually accused you of anything or criticized you. You are 'projecting' your insecurities onto others.

Denial

People in denial refuse to accept the reality of a fact or experience. It is a way of protecting our self-esteem to fail to acknowledge or own our behaviour or an experience. Denial may be used by victims of trauma or people in fearful situations, and may even be a beneficial initial protective response. In the long run, however, denial prevents you from processing and acknowledging unpleasant information about yourself, or about your involvement with other people, and can have potentially destructive consequences.

'I didn't see anyone get hurt.'
'I've never laid a finger on anyone in my life!'
'What are you talking about? I barely drink these days. I haven't touched a drop in months.'
'What are you on about? I'm not aggressive.'
'I was only doing my job.'

Displacement

'Displacement' is a term used to suggest a defence mechanism whereby the mind operates unconsciously to transfer emotions, ideas or wishes onto someone else to allay anxiety in the face of aggressive impulses. An example is scapegoating, where aggression may be displaced onto people with little or no connection with what is causing anger. A young man kicks the wheel of his car after an argument with his girlfriend; a woman snaps at her housemate when she is upset about something that happened at work that day. Displacement can become a chain reaction, with people unwittingly becoming both targets of displacement and perpetrators of it. For example, a man is angry after feeling belittled and insulted by his supervisor at work, but he cannot express this so at home he hits his wife. The wife hits one of the children, possibly disguising this as punishment (rationalization). The child lashes out at his younger sibling and so on.

> 'What did I tell you about leaving the milk out of the fridge? You're so selfish, Mary! Now we'll have to chuck it out and there'll be none for tomorrow's breakfast!'
>
> 'Hey, Sam, don't have a go at me just because you had a bad day! I am sick of you coming home and having a go at me. Billy, stop that racket, do you hear?'
>
> Their son Billy is shouting at the dog to 'Drop!' (the dog has a piece of his Lego in his mouth), but on getting a ticking off from his mum he takes a swipe at the dog. 'I hate you, Rex, you stupid dog!'

Overt aggression

Overt aggression involves outward or open confrontational acts of aggression, such as physical fighting, violence, verbal threats and bullying.

Scenario 1

In a real-life online case, when the rapper 'Dolla' (Roderick Anthony Burton II) was shot in May 2009 a British troll left racist remarks and derogatory comments on his RIP tribute on Facebook. The same internet troll performed a similar callous act on Boxing Day 2011 when a university student was murdered. The day after his death the troll left an offensive comment on the student's Facebook RIP tribute page. It read, 'Rot in piss.'

Scenario 2
A 20-year-old male randomly attacked a stranger while he was waiting in a queue for a bus. The victim was hit so hard that he was forced through the doors of the newly arrived bus. When a teenager attempted to tend to the victim the perpetrator told him to leave it because 'the piece of s*** deserved it'.

Scenario 3
Harry was in a supermarket peering into a freezer cabinet for a bag of frozen chips when someone's trolley rammed into the back of his legs.

'Look where you're going, you f***ing idiot,' slurred a heavily built and intoxicated man.

'You look where you're going, you mean, you t**t!' Harry replied.

The man thrust the trolley towards Harry again and this time it hit him so hard it upturned and its contents – mostly cans of lager – clanged and scattered about the supermarket floor.

'You jerk, what'd you do that for? You f***ing w****r!' shouted Harry.

Things escalated; the man took a wild swing at Harry, but missed and fell to the floor.

A few minutes later help was at hand and the man was escorted out of the supermarket by two security officers.

Passive aggression

Is there someone in your life who makes you feel like you are on an emotional roller coaster? Do you know a person who is friendly one minute, but sulks and withdraws the next? Does a family member or friend consistently procrastinate, postpone, stall and shut down any difficult conversation, especially if it is about how he or she upset you? Steve (the character mentioned in Chapter 1) is a very passive person like this who avoids confrontation at all costs. Anne is his wife of 18 years. To counter Anne's annoyance at his antics and passivity, increasingly he gives her the silent treatment.

Common passive aggressive strategies include:

- being ambiguous in order to create confusion;
- making chronic excuses for lack of follow-through or poor performance;
- creating drama or chaotic situations;
- procrastinating, particularly at the expense of others so as to annoy them;
- being chronically late or intentionally 'forgetting' things in order to control or punish;

- avoiding intimacy;
- using guilt or sulking to punish or gain attention;
- blaming others for mistakes or conflict;
- creating intentional obstructions to punish or get one's own way;
- being argumentative or critical in order to get one's own way;
- being unresponsive or non-communicative to avoid discomfort or conflict;
- withholding kindness, love, or actions (such as sex or household tasks or favours);
- sabotaging (either overtly or covertly) the efforts or relationships of others.

Phrases expressed by passive aggressive people include:

'Sure. Whatever.'
'I'm not angry, whatever gave you that idea?'
'Fine. Do what you want!'

Going off in a huff or withdrawing from arguments are core strategies of the passive aggressive person. Since passive aggression is motivated by a person's belief that expressing anger directly will only make life worse, the passive aggressive person uses phrases such as these to express anger to shut down communication, to avoid confronting emotions he or she most likely doesn't want to acknowledge in him- or herself, let alone in other people.

People who habitually engage in passive aggressive behaviour often verbally comply with a request, but behaviourally delay its completion.

'I am coming. Why are you always so impatient?'
'I said I would do it. I don't have to jump when you say jump. I'll do it when I can find the time.'
'Why are you so annoyed with me? I said I would do it, didn't I?'
'You never said I had to do it today!'

When these strategies and exchanges lead to hostility being aired, the passive aggressive individual tends to withdraw from the situation or give the other person the silent treatment.

Covert aggression

Covert aggression is the opposite of passive aggression in that, though it is concealed, there is nothing passive about it! It is very active aggression. Covert aggressive personalities are the archetypal wolves in sheep's clothing, according to the psychologist and author George Simon, who wrote the book *In Sheep's Clothing.*[7] Being the target of a covert aggressive person can be a traumatic experience. In an earlier book, *The Empathy Trap* (Sheldon Press, 2013), the covert aggression and antics of antisocial personalities such as sociopaths are described. The experience can make a person feel as if he or she is going crazy.

Scenario 1
Elizabeth is a professional woman at the height of her career. With a comfortable lifestyle, a loving husband and beautiful daughter, she felt she had it all. That was until the day she made the shocking discovery that her husband of 25 years had been conning her. Without her knowing, over several years he had racked up enormous debt. He had hidden this by drawing down a 'salary' from one of the couple's joint accounts to keep up the pretence that he had an income. One day while speaking to the mortgage company Elizabeth learned that he had forged her name on a second mortgage. She called him from work to ask him what was going on, but he hung up on her, then left the family home without explanation or apology and no way to contact him. Elizabeth was left in a traumatized and shocked state. It took her a long time to pick up the pieces.

Scenario 2
From her first day working for the company, Julie charmed the pants off her seniors and sucked up to anyone with influence. She was confident and gained a reputation as a high achiever.

Behind the scenes, and unbeknown to anyone, she was stealing office equipment. One day, however, Julie became aware that one of her colleagues had suspicions, so she set about laying the blame elsewhere. She reported the laptop from her office stolen and spread malicious gossip about the staff member who had suspicions about her.

Two months later, Julie resigned from her job. Everyone congratulated her and wished her success with her new venture, a consultancy business! Unfortunately for all, and especially for the colleague who had been alert to her ruses and seen her reputation sullied, Julie got away with it.

Strategies commonly used by online aggressors

Covert aggression is also seen in online communication. It can be veiled as humour. People who engage in it often use sarcasm to put down or belittle the other person. They also tend to avoid emotional situations. It is not a self-enhancing way of communicating and is often used by people who have low self-esteem who generally want to keep people at bay. It is used to confirm to the individual that engaging in communication with other people is a waste of time and energy.

There is a shortage of research concerning the issue of online trolling. According to a leading researcher on the language of aggression, Dr Claire Hardaker of Lancaster University, 'trolling' is a term used to describe online antagonism that dates back to the 1980s. It is deliberate antagonism undertaken for amusement's sake.

At their most extreme, trolls are everyday sadists or people with personality disorders, such as ASPD. The techniques used blend with gaslighting, as mentioned earlier, and can cause manifold problems for the targeted person, not least high anxiety, fear and distress. This is commonly termed cyberbullying.

'Cyberbullying' has been defined as repeated harm inflicted through the use of computers and other electronic devices. This behaviour may involve the sending of harassing messages, the making of derogatory comments on a website, or intimidating or threatening someone in various online settings of public forums, video games, blogs, or social networking sites. Cyberbullying does not necessarily imply a personal relationship where the victim and instigator know each other, as would be assumed in bullying in the real world.

In recent years an increasing number of cases of cyberbullicide, which describes suicide indirectly or directly influenced by experiences of online aggression, have been reported in the mass media. Most of these involve teenagers, who take their own lives as a result of being harassed and mistreated over the internet.

Findings of online aggression research by Adam Zimmerman suggest that although anonymity may increase the likelihood that individuals will act aggressively, social modelling influences aggressive outcomes.[8] Zimmerman draws attention to the process of dehumanization, where certain social conditions reduce an individual's self-awareness and concern about what other people feel or even think about them. This process weakens the restraints against the expression of undesirable behaviour. He cites a 1970s study by

Philip George Zimbardo, a psychologist and emeritus professor at Stanford University – the infamous Stanford prison experiment. In the study individuals who were dressed in guard uniforms and glasses to hide their faces and identity engaged in cruel behaviours towards prisoners that presumably would not have occurred had they not been anonymous. Zimbardo, in a *New York Times* interview in 2007, suggested that 'when someone is anonymous it opens the door to all kinds of antisocial behaviour'. Claire Hardaker has studied the language of aggression and describes some common strategies used by online aggressors below.[9]

- **Digression** involves straying from the purpose of the discussion or forum. It includes malicious spamming, or introducing entirely irrelevant topics.
- **(Hypo)criticism** involves criticizing others, usually excessively, for an offence of which the critic is also guilty. The word is derived from hypocrite, hypocritical.
- **Antipathy** involves proactively and usually covertly exploiting a sensitive discussion by being deliberately controversial or provocative.
- **Endangering** involves masquerading as help or advice giver while actually causing harm.
- **Shock** involves being insensitive or explicit about a sensitive or taboo topic such as religion, death, politics, human rights, animal welfare – a classic strategy.
- **Aggress** involves openly and deliberately aggressing another person, without any clear justification and with the aim of antagonizing him or her into retaliating.

3

Dealing with aggression without being aggressive

> Most of us think of ourselves as thinking creatures that feel, but we are actually feeling creatures that think.
>
> Jill Bolte Taylor (neuroanatomist)

In the previous chapter different sorts of aggressive behaviour that people are exposed to in everyday life were highlighted. If we respond in kind, by becoming aggressive ourselves, then more often than not the situation and aggression soon escalate. This chapter looks at what can be done to deal with aggressive people non-aggressively as we go about our daily lives. In subsequent chapters, I shall provide practical tips on how to formulate non-aggressive responses after being on the receiving end of different sorts of aggression.

What can we do to help ourselves?

To help ourselves become more aware of aggression in ourselves as well as in other people, we need to increase our sensitive awareness of our surroundings and other people. We need to make use of our moral-emotion apparatus, an outcome of which can see us empathize with other people as opposed to feeling hostile towards them. Empathy is the experience of understanding other people's perspectives – you place yourself in their shoes and feel what they are feeling. Empathizing helps us survive everyday life for it helps us to gauge appropriate responses to other people in social situations.

In Chapter 2, the idea was introduced that we each have a default position along the empathy spectrum and are positioned somewhere from zero empathy to high empathy (see Table 1, p. 21). Most of us have middling abilities as far as empathy goes, which means that we can be swayed in either direction when we face fear-making situations: towards empathic action or towards indifference and apathy to other people or even ourselves.

When faced with a threat of aggression or violence, our survival apparatus kicks in. For those who are 'instinct intact', this means that we prepare to fight or take flight, but some of us are 'instinct injured', meaning we cannot locate feelings within to alert us about dangerous situations or encounters. If this early warning system is not in good working order, we may find ourselves unable to determine a course of action to help ourselves get out of harm's way. In some people, their difficulty in locating and processing feelings is so marked that it affects their emotional awareness, social attachment and interpersonal relating. Furthermore, they may have difficulty in distinguishing and appreciating the emotions of others, which is thought to lead to ineffective emotional responding.

Moral-emotion apparatus

It rarely pays to take a hostile stance when confronted with aggression, because more often than not the situation escalates, along with the threat of hostility and violence. Nor does it usually pay to remain impassive to one's own or another's plight in the face of a threat. Playing dead, as some animals do (this is called 'tonic immobility' and is a natural state of paralysis or hypnosis), may be a way of avoiding or deterring predators to get out of a dangerous situation, but it cannot be maintained in the long term.

So what can we do to help ourselves? There are actions we can take that can influence our responses to other people. As outlined in Chapter 2, all of us use our moral-emotion apparatus to influence and guide our actions. Some of us use this apparatus more often and to better effect than others. Nevertheless, apart from those who are extremely antisocial – people with zero empathy whose traits are fixed by adulthood – most of us can improve and exercise our moral-emotion apparatus and put it to good use.

Using our moral-emotion apparatus requires utilizing our empathic abilities. It also involves the ability to reflect on our own conduct and making use of moral feelings to shape and guide our actions. Empathy is a process that leads to expression of behaviour that is socially beneficial. In essence, empathizing is the process by which we engage in pro-social activity.

In his book *The Age of Empathy*, primatologist Frans de Waal argues that our greatest hope for building a fairer society is based on a more generous and accurate view of human nature. Being in tune with others, he notes, are traits linked to empathy that produce the glue which holds communities together.[1] So how is empathy and the process of empathizing defined? The answers to this question are explored next.

Cognitive empathy

'Cognitive empathy' is knowing how other people feel and what they might be thinking. This is sometimes called 'perspective-taking'.

There can be a dark side to this sort of empathy. In fact, those who fall within the 'dark triad' – narcissists, psychopaths and Machiavellians (see Chapter 2) – possess this ability, while having no emotional concern whatever for their victims.

Affective or emotional empathy

Affective or emotional empathy is when you feel along with the other person. Emotional empathy enables us to tune into another person's inner emotional world. Our own experience of feelings (feeling sad, happy, outraged and so on) helps us to feel along with the other person. If our range of feelings is limited (for example, a sociopath's feelings may be restricted to base feelings such as anger, envy and self-pity), we may have difficulty recognizing feelings in others that we don't readily access or process in ourselves. Conversely, a highly sensitive person may have an expansive emotional range to draw on to aid him or her in emotionally empathizing with other people.

One downside of emotional empathy is when people lack the ability to manage their own distressing emotions. This can lead to emotional exhaustion and distress. Doctors and healthcare workers often employ purposeful detachment in order to protect themselves against stress and burnout. They use their cognitive empathic skills, as opposed to their emotional empathy, to aid them in their work with patients. Of course, there is a danger that employing emotional detachment can lead to indifference, rather than well-regulated caring. Those who work with people in need – whose business it is to show care and concern for others – have to find ways to maintain a healthy balance in order to provide compassionate care. What this takes is emotional intelligence and the wherewithal to manage emotions in a self-enhancing way.

Emotional intelligence

As we emotionally mature through childhood and into adulthood, we learn and take on board moral standards that we absorb from the individuals around us, from society at large and the people who make up the community we live in. All being well, the development of these moral standards passes through several stages during childhood and adolescence, moving from avoidance of punishment to avoidance of disapproval and rejection, then finally avoidance of guilt and self-recrimination. Unfortunately, some people dodge the last step in the process.

All emotions are impulses to act. The emotions of fear, anger, happiness, love, surprise, disgust and sadness send signals to the brain that release hormones to give strength to the necessary reactions. Being alert to our feelings is important to thought, and vice versa, and emotional thought leads to action for coping and surviving. Hence humans are of two minds: the 'emotional mind' and the 'rational mind'. One mind feels and the other thinks.

Of course, these two minds interact. Emotion is known to influence thought in many ways. It informs the rational mind, which moderates the involvement and expression of our emotions. This said, some of us have greater access to our feelings and a more expansive emotional range than others, so there is considerable individual variation. In the emotional mind is lodged impulsive, powerful and often illogical feelings, while the rational mind affords us the ability to think and reflect. This supports the view of neuroanatomist Jill Bolte Taylor, quoted at the start of the chapter – we are actually 'feeling creatures that think'.

The concept of 'emotional intelligence' emerged in psychological research and constitutes three components of the mind: cognition (thought), affect (feeling) and motivation. To make use of one's emotions in an intelligent way requires us to connect the first two components of the mind: cognition and feeling. The theory of emotional intelligence links cognition and feeling by suggesting that emotions make cognitive processes more intelligent and that one can think intelligently about emotions. Emotional intelligence is defined as the ability to:

- perceive accurately, appraise and express emotion;
- generate and access feelings when they facilitate thought;

- understand emotions and emotional knowledge;
- regulate emotions in order to promote emotional and intellectual growth.[2]

People who are aware of their own and others' emotions gain a large amount of information about themselves and their environment. For example, a singer who is sensitive to experiencing pre-performance anxiety will know that she needs to find ways to keep calm before she goes on stage. Over time she learns to manage this situation so that it does not affect her actual performance. Individuals who do not recognize their own and others' emotions are cut off from this useful information.

Understanding feelings involves having a language of emotion with which to express our understanding of our felt experiences. People feel sadness after experiencing some sort of loss, for example, and feel happiness after experiencing a gain.

Emotional intelligence and management combine to help us understand how emotions merge together (for instance, that we can experience feelings such as anger and disgust at the same time) and how they change over time in given situations (for example, bereavement is a process that can see us experience at different times shock and emotional numbness, anger and sadness). Management of emotion refers to the ability to regulate one's own emotions. Some techniques for managing emotions work more effectively than others. For instance, using alcohol as a way to cope with intense feelings of grief is usually not an effective way to deal with grief; it temporarily blocks the experience of intense feeling, but in the end we have to face and accept our loss. Permitting rather than blocking the full sweep of emotional experience is probably the best way for us to come to terms with loss.

Emotion management consequently involves two important processes. It involves both knowing what strategies are most effective and expressing emotions appropriately. It does not entail ignoring or suppressing feelings. On the contrary, experiencing a range of feelings and expressing them can be useful and indeed helpful (for example, in coming to terms with loss). Feelings are, then, best viewed as indicators of our state of being, as opposed to 'good' and 'bad' experiences.

Instincts, intuition and survival

Humans are born with, and also acquire along the way, a toolbox of strategies and social impulses to survive. In terms of how we live our daily lives, humans have two very different systems in relation to the way we operate. One system is our instinctual and often subconscious way of operating. The second is more analytical.

The word 'instinct' derives from *instinctus* or 'impulse' and is the innate inclination towards a particular behaviour in response to certain stimuli. It is instinctive in us to recognize when to run from a perceived danger. This is known as the 'fight or flight' response, as previously mentioned.

The word 'intuition' dates back to late Middle English, when it denoted spiritual insight or immediate spiritual communication. It derives from the Latin *intueri*, meaning 'consider'. It is the automatic thought process that doesn't require analysis. The intuitive system is more hardwired into the human species than commonly understood. Unfortunately, such gut feelings can also be silenced and suppressed. A childhood hijacked by abusive or neglectful people can make it difficult to separate traumatic past experiences from gut intuition or instinct. And strong emotions, particularly negative ones, can cloud our intuition. A person's intuition may fail when he or she is depressed or angry or in a heightened emotional state.

The main thing that distinguishes intuitive people is that they listen to their intuitions and gut feelings, rather than ignore them. Most of us, if not all, are connected to our intuition, but some people don't pay attention to it. There is growing interest in how individuals can learn to use our intuitive cognition. By way of example, in 2012 the *New York Times* reported that the United States Navy planned to start a programme to investigate how members of the military can be trained to improve their intuitive ability. The idea came from the testimony of troops in Iraq and Afghanistan who reported an unexplained feeling of danger just before they encountered an enemy attack or ran into an improvised explosive device.

A new language and approach for dealing with aggression

Why are many of us so accommodating and nice in daily life? Often what belies niceness in the face of hostility is fear – fear of conflict. Permitting others to be offensive or aggressive, however, gives the message that they are entitled to treat us this way. If someone is rude to you, you should not feel obligated to put up with it.

We need to learn when to speak up and when to stay silent. We need to speak up if our silence could be damaging – emotionally or physically – to ourselves or to other people. We should stay silent if what we seek is revenge, for example, because retaliation tends to lead to an escalation of aggression and violence.

Psychiatrist Marcia Sirota has an approach that is helpful in dealing with aggressive people. She is the originator of the concept 'ruthless compassion' and founder of the Ruthless Compassion Institute. So what is ruthless compassion? Dr Sirota says it is many things, but, distilled down, it is about being responsible for yourself and your choices and holding yourself accountable for your actions. It is about freedom from duty; you act on what you know is right, rather than what you think you 'should' do, or what you think others want you to do. You do what's right, but not at your own expense. Ruthless compassion allows freedom from self-criticism and self-doubt and, especially, freedom from the fear of other people's judgements. You see yourself clearly and make corrections as you go. You want to connect with others, but you're not preoccupied with pleasing them or afraid of displeasing them. Ruthless compassion is letting go of the need for approval or acceptance from others, speaking your truth even if it isn't popular, believing in yourself and trusting yourself, being courageous and having integrity. It is about listening to your inner wisdom (all the accumulated data that you take in subconsciously each day, over many years) and trusting your intuition about the people and situations you encounter; it's not being a cynic but, rather, a healthy sceptic; it's questioning the status quo; it's going after what you want as opposed to running from what you fear. It is having clear, firm boundaries, without being rigid or unreasonable; it's knowing how to simply say 'no' and disengage from drama.

'Rolling with resistance' is a technique borrowed from the field of behaviour change (in particular the work of two psychologists, Bill Miller and Stephen Rollnick)[3] which recognizes that simply attacking or confronting someone directly does not always work. In fact, it may lead people to be highly defensive or confrontational. If you can remember a situation where you yourself were feeling attacked or criticized, you might recognize how defensive this made you feel. Outlined are some of the ways in which we can roll with resistance instead of being confrontational or attacking in response to hostility. I will apply some of these techniques and ideas in subsequent chapters, where I take a practical look at responding to overt, passive and covert aggression and hostility without becoming hostile ourselves.

- Reflect back, in a neutral way, what people say. If what is being said is exaggerated or unreasonable, then simply hearing the words relayed back to them without being attacked may prompt them to tone it down. If people expect you to criticize them, a simple restatement of their views may disarm them.
- Amplify aggressors' unreasonableness and hostility. Expose it so that they and other people who bear witness can hear it, too. Usually aggressors will attempt to impression manage the situation if there is an audience and will calm down.
- Emphasize personal choice. Make it clear that it is the aggressors' decision and choice how they deal with conflict.
- If you're expected to respond to people's hostile attacks, ask them what they are upset about, in order to show that you are interested in communicating rather than arguing.
- You can defend yourself without adopting a defensive tone: 'It is true that I made a mistake.' Stand up for yourself by reiterating the specific error, but refuse to accept rudeness and offensive comment.
- Demonstrate a willingness to understand difficult people's frustrations without blame or defensiveness: 'You seem angry about this and I'm sorry about that.'
- Resist the urge to fight to win the argument. Listening and asking questions leads others to their own better conclusions.

Standing up for ourselves and others

As mentioned in Chapter 2, in the 1960s Professor Milgram of Yale University set out to test the human propensity to obey orders. In the experiment, a participant in the role of 'teacher' was asked to administer an electric shock to the 'learner' whenever he or she answered a question incorrectly, with the voltage gradually increasing each time. In the experiments, 65 per cent of participants administered what they thought was the experiment's final massive 450-volt shock. Milgram's experiments were said to show that few people, when asked to carry out actions incompatible with fundamental standards of morality, have the resources needed to resist authority. A new study by sociologist Matthew Hollander takes a different stance, however, looking at the different acts of resistance to the authority figure (the teacher) shown by Milgram's participants.[4] This isn't the first time researchers have explored defiance in the Milgram paradigm, but it's the most comprehensive analysis of resistance strategies as revealed through the dialogue in Milgram's original studies.

Hollander identified a number of implicit and explicit forms of resistance to authority figures. Here are the explicit ones.

- Personalizing the situation (such as in the case of the experiment, the learner was asked if he was happy to continue with the test).
- Prompting domineering people and questioning the ethical nature of their commands, especially if their requests are that you do something to another person that seems unethical (in the case of the experiment, the command was challenged because the learner was in obvious pain).
- 'Stop tries', in which the participant stated that he did not want to continue in the experiment. In real life, this would be equivalent to saying, 'No! I won't take part in this bullying or act of aggression.'

Hollander suggests that these findings may provide ways to improve our understanding of the interpersonal dynamics of authority and resistance to authority in order to save lives and empower individuals (whether bystanders or victims) when presented with overbearing individuals, such as when they are in situations of sexual harassment and intimidation.

Just how realistic is it to see real reductions in the aggression we experience, specifically in light of increasing online communication, which is so easily influenced by the power and influence of social modelling? Over the course of the following chapters, I suggest practical ways to counter aggression in daily life. Behaviours may well be socially infectious, but if we each take responsibility for doing our bit to reduce our own aggression, then we have a chance of seeing some reduction in culture.

4

Weathering hostility

In the Aesop's fable 'The Oak and the Reeds', the reeds pride themselves on being able to bow and yield to every breeze so that the
gale passes harmlessly over their heads, unlike the oak tree, which
is torn up by the roots and hurled into the river. Like the reeds in
the fable, we benefit from an approach and way of communicating
that enables us to survive the tempestuous. In this chapter, I discuss
how to respond effectively to aggression without becoming aggressive yourself. I offer practical tips intended to help you establish
a new style of communication – one that enables you to communicate assertively and maintain good boundaries. Of course, each
of us has our own mode of expression and way of putting things.
These examples, which can be adapted to suit, illustrate how shifts
in language and approach can bring about better outcomes when
dealing with hostility in everyday life.

Table 2 outlines the different positions we take when interacting
with other people. These ideas are drawn from the 1967 book by
Thomas A. Harris, *I'm OK, You're OK*, one of the bestselling self-help
books ever published. Here I give an abridged version of Harris's
identified positions (his fourth position is not included, however –
'I'm not OK, you're not OK' – as this is less common, although it
can arise in children and adults who have been abused). The position
in the middle column – 'I'm OK, you're OK' – is your best bet for
maintaining an assertive stance. Although we tend to fall back on one
position, that position can alter depending on the people we're interacting with. For example, if the person we are communicating with
is domineering, we may unintentionally become meeker; if the other
person is passive, we may find ourselves becoming more dominant.

Initiating boundaries

Initiating and upholding personal boundaries provides a way to
show hostile people that we won't tolerate their antics. This is

Table 2 'I'm OK, you're OK'

You're OK, I'm not	I'm OK, you're OK	I'm OK, you're not
Belief Your view is more important than my own, so it doesn't matter what I think	**Belief** I believe and act as if we both deserve respect. We are equally entitled to have things done our way	**Belief** I believe I am entitled to have things done my way, because I am right. You are wrong and not entitled to do things your way
Consequences This person gives in to others, doesn't get what he or she wants or needs and has self-critical thoughts	**Consequences** This person generally has good relationships, is happy to compromise, but doesn't disregard his or her own wants and needs	**Consequences** This person often upsets others and him- or herself and often feels angry and resentful

ruthless compassion in action. The aggressor may operate along the lines of, 'I have been hurt, so it's OK to hurt you', but if you say something such as, 'I don't have to tolerate this aggression from you', it may well serve as a reminder of what is really going on in the exchange.

If we habitually let people stand close and get personal or direct offensive comments at us or we put up with physical abuse, all this says to the aggressor is, 'I will let you hurt me because I need to avoid conflict'. It won't stop that person behaving aggressively. This is even more likely to happen if the aggressor lacks self-awareness or a conscience, which makes it important that you impose boundaries of communication and some safe distance between the agressor and you.

Personal boundaries are the limits we establish to protect ourselves from being manipulated, used or violated by other people. They include material boundaries (money, clothes, food), physical boundaries (your personal space, privacy and body) and mental boundaries (your thoughts, values and opinions). Emotional boundaries distinguish separating your emotions and responsibility for them from someone else's; sexual boundaries protect your comfort level with sexual activity – what, where, when and with whom; and internal boundaries involve regulating your relationship with yourself. Learning to manage negative thoughts and feelings empowers you, as does the ability to follow through on goals and those commitments you've made to yourself. Last, but most important, boundaries help us express our individuality.

Boundaries can be learned

Not all of us are shown during childhood how to maintain healthy boundaries, but the good news is that boundaries can be learned if we see the value and importance of them in our lives. It helps if you are able to do the kinds of things described below.

- You know that you have a right and also a responsibility to put into effect personal boundaries. Your boundaries demonstrate what is acceptable in your life and what is not.
- You can recognize that other people's needs and feelings are not more important than your own.
- You are able and willing to say 'no' when something doesn't feel right. Many of us put ourselves at a disadvantage by trying to accommodate other people – even people who violate our boundaries.
- You are able to identify the conduct and behaviours that you find unacceptable. Let others know when they have overstepped your boundaries. Do not be afraid to tell other people what actions you may need to take if your wishes are not respected.
- You trust yourself and care about what you need, want and value.

Taking cues from your feelings

Anger often is a signal that action is required. If you feel resentful or attacked and are blaming someone for the situation you find yourself in, it might mean that you haven't been setting boundaries. If you feel anxious or guilty about setting boundaries, remind yourself that your relationships suffer when you don't. Although it might seem a tall order at first to instigate boundaries, once you practise setting boundaries, you will more than likely soon feel empowered. It takes time, support and relearning to be able to set effective boundaries. Self-awareness and taking cues from your feelings helps.

Confronting hostility without being hostile

A lot of people cannot handle confrontation and are fearful of it. They lose control of their voice pitch and may feel the urge to hit out. This is the 'fight or flight' syndrome kicking in, which pumps adrenaline throughout your body in readiness either to kick back or to run away from someone you think might harm you. Hostility and aggression come in many forms, some of which are listed below, with definitions.

- **Discounting** to disregard what people say or do and treat them as unworthy of consideration; to pay no attention to, take no notice of, take no account of, overlook, dismiss, ignore.
- **Intimidating** to deliberately frighten, menace, terrify, scare, alarm, terrorize or unnerve someone.
- **Belittling** to dismiss someone or some situation as unimportant; disparage, denigrate, run down, deprecate, depreciate, play down, trivialize, minimize, undervalue.
- **Excluding** to deny someone access to a place, group or privilege; ban, prohibit, reject, ostracize, freeze out, send to Coventry.
- **Manipulating** to control or influence people or situations in an unscrupulous way; to deliberately exploit, seek to control, influence and use/turn to one's advantage, manoeuvre, engineer situations and 'manage' the people involved. For instance, you make a statement and someone turns it around to be used against you in a negative way. He or she says something offensive about you, but later denies it, then makes you feel guilty or says you are oversensitive. Manipulators are indirect and take the passive aggressive route.
- **Violence** to use physical force intended to hurt, damage or kill someone or something; brutality, cruelty.

Hostility needs to be dealt with, but the nature of the hostility will affect the nature of your response. Clearly, in extreme cases of violence, it is necessary to act fast to protect oneself and get away.

Dealing with violent people

- If you can avoid dealing with a violent person, do so. If you fear you are physically in danger, call the emergency services immediately. Let the police handle those situations.
- If you need to deal with a violent person such as a friend or partner who is not trying to physically hurt you, try to calm him or her down. Talk to your partner calmly and clearly. Let your partner know how he or she is acting right now and try to let your partner tell you what the problem is. It is very important

that, whatever you do, you try not to yell at the violent person; yelling will only aggravate your partner and may cause him or her to act even more violently and defensively.

- If the violent person is trying to physically hurt you, get out of the situation as and when you can and call the emergency services straight away. It is OK to run from the situation. You can fight back, but only to protect yourself or in a life or death situation.
- If your partner is physically abusive, you need to get out of the relationship immediately. If that's impossible without getting violent yourself, then seek shelter. Frequently in cases of domestic violence an abusive partner will justify the violence in his or her mind. Often emotional manipulation is involved, so do not believe it if your partner tells you how sorry he or she is after having hurt you. If your partner really loves you, he or she will never try to hurt you.
- Almost all abusive partners will stay abusive. Even if your partner shows remorse and the abuse seems to stop for a while, so you think he or she has changed, unfortunately, the day will soon come when the anger and rage will erupt again.
- Do not get caught up in the violence and start acting violently yourself. You have to show the person with violent tendencies that being violent doesn't solve anything and let him or her know you don't accept violent behaviour from anyone.
- It is very hard for people to change what they have thought was OK for their whole lives. Violence can become an entrenched pattern of behaviour. You should consider and make plans to get away, and stay away, from people for whom violence is a way of life.
- Do get help. It would be dreadful if you ended up severely hurt and no one had any idea what was going on with you. Friends can help, but you need to give them the opportunity, so find the courage to talk of your experiences.

Dealing with verbal hostility

In many other situations there are alternatives to being someone's punchbag or striking back. The first thing to notice is how we are feeling in the moment and in dealing with the situation. Give yourself pause for thought and take note of what you feel. Is what the person is saying making you feel defensive, anxious, fearful, angry or mad? Ask yourself not if you or the other person is right, but do you like being treated the way you are being treated? If not, then it is time to assert yourself and establish some clear boundaries.

From the position of 'I'm OK, you're OK', you aim to act as if both of you deserve respect; you are both equally entitled to have things done your way. You maintain this stance even if the other person fits the 'you're OK, I'm not' position – often adopted by individuals who are passive aggressive – or even the 'I'm OK, you're not' position – the stance of the heavy-handed and authoritarian. Maintaining a respectful line of communication and the 'I'm OK, you're OK' position enables you to assert yourself, while amplifying the other person's unreasonableness and hostility. Below is an approach you could consider taking, with some example responses included.

1 **What is going on?** Once you have paused for thought and listened to the other person's rant, you may want to assert a boundary and ask what is going on to cause the evolving situation.

    'Sorry?'
    'Why are you shouting at me?'
    'I don't understand what this is about.'
    'What are you saying?'
    'Why are you being so aggressive?'
    'I am confused.'

    This turns the focus back on the aggressive person for a minute, which might calm him or her down as a lot of people get lost in the moment and don't realize they are being aggressive.

2 **Identify the problem** This gives the person who is hostile or angry a chance to explain his or her view, while giving you the chance to take stock of the situation.

    'Is something wrong?'
    'You are angry because you think I did something wrong?'

    Don't get sucked into such arguments. The other person's purpose is to make sure you lose the argument, thereby showing that he or she has won. If you don't get sucked in there is no argument to win.

3 **Problem-solve** Show that you are willing to see this from the other person's perspective. Without accepting blame, see if he or she will attempt to resolve the issue.

'I am sorry, I didn't realize.'
'I am glad you told me.'
'Let's try and solve this.'
'Let's see if we can find a way of resolving this.'

4 **Amplify the other person's unreasonableness** Reflect the unreasonableness and lack of willingness to resolve the problem. This can help in situations where there is an audience or bystanders, where you need help and witnesses.

'You don't want to find a way forward?'
'You are not concerned how I feel about this?'
'It is OK for you to get want you want, even if I lose out?'
'So it doesn't matter how I feel about this?'
'I am willing to find a way to resolve this in a way that works for us both.'

5 **Lay down the boundary** At some point we have to stand up to aggressors to leave them in no doubt that their behaviour is unacceptable.

'This is unacceptable.'
'I will not agree to that.'
'I am not sure that we can go any further with this if you are not willing to work this out together.'
'If you are not willing to work with me towards a way to resolve this, I will take this forward as a complaint of harassment.'
'If you change your mind and you think we can find a way to resolve this, I'd be happy to hear from you.'

In subsequent chapters I discuss ways of putting these ideas, values and principles into action when dealing with specific types of aggression, beginning with passive aggression in Chapter 5.

5

Dealing with passive aggression

Behaving in a passive aggressive way does not mean that you are a bad person. Often it's a strategy used by people who are afraid to be honest and open. Whether we ourselves are passive aggressive, or we are dealing with other people's passive aggression, the resulting behaviour can be very challenging and can test and strain relationships. In this chapter I look at how to recognize it and counter it in everyday life.

Passive aggression was first defined during the Second World War to describe soldiers who were not openly defiant, but expressed a lack of compliance through passive measures, such as pouting, stubbornness, procrastination and passive obstruction. These behaviours were thought of as immaturity and a reaction to the stress and discipline of military life.

Passive aggressive behaviour is the indirect expression of hostility. It often manifests as procrastination, sullenness, or as failure to accomplish requested tasks. Passive aggression is a learned way of responding to other people. It can arise and be a consequence of growing up in an environment with strict social rules and little opportunity to express one's individuality. If it continues past adolescence and into adulthood, passive aggression becomes a form of resistance and a reaction to being unable to express one's feelings and thoughts freely.

Passive aggression gets in the way of positive relationships. Those who exhibit passive aggression are full of unacknowledged contradictions, such as compliant defiance and hostile cooperation, and people interacting with them may find this confusing and upsetting. People with such tendencies don't tend to let others know how they really feel or what they really want. Passive aggression provides a way and means for them to avoid uncomfortable feelings and situations. Being uneasy with honest conversation and often on the defensive means, however, that the person with passive aggressive tendencies will frequently mistake honest and respectful dialogue with others as criticism and personal attack.

Examples of passive aggressive behaviour

Confrontational style of questioning

Although it seems paradoxical, people who exhibit passive aggression often respond to other people in a confrontational and threat-based way. It is a defensive mechanism and a projection of their own unacceptable qualities. Projection is a defence mechanism that involves taking our own unacceptable qualities or feelings and ascribing them to other people. For example, if you dislike or resent someone, you might instead believe that that person resents or dislikes you. This style of questioning tends to put the other person on the defensive. For example:

> 'What are you, a psychic? You don't know what I'm thinking!'
> 'I am *not* defensive. Why are *you* so defensive?'
> 'Why on earth would you even think that?'
> 'What's wrong with you?'
> 'Why do you have a go at me all the time?'
> 'Why do you make out I don't do anything to help around here?'

Veiled put-downs and insults

Another, far less benign approach of the passive aggressive is to make use of put-downs and insults. For example:

> 'I wish I could work full time and be career-minded like you, but I think children need their mother at home.'
> 'I wish I had the luxury of working from home. You must have so much leisure time. Personally I wouldn't know what to do with myself!'
> 'Oh, you've lost some weight. You definitely needed to. My, you were fat!'
> 'Where am I going on holiday? Some of us have too much to do and too little time to take holidays!'
> 'Some of us have family to take care of and can't go swanning around pleasing ourselves!'

'Whatever! My opinion doesn't count anyway. You'll do what you like regardless. You always do.'

Comments like these (often intentional), including sarcastic humour, are targeted at a specific individual and intended to make the receiver feel guilty for getting or doing whatever it is that the person making the comments cannot.

Indirect violence

The passive aggressive person may engage in indirect acts of violence such as destruction of property or slamming doors, all in the sight of another person. The point of this sort of behaviour is that they want you to know that they are angry and/or frustrated.

Withholding support and affection

Ignoring phone calls, emails or texts from friends and loved ones is another way in which passive aggressive individuals signal that they are upset. Instead of communicating clearly and honestly, the person with passive aggressive tendencies punishes friends and relations with the silent treatment or cold shoulder. This can extend to other areas of relationship and disrupt daily life if the individual refrains from undertaking roles and tasks they are personally responsible for, or they withhold support or affection.

Catastrophizing

People who dislike intense feelings and struggle to express them appropriately may displace their anger onto other people or even inanimate objects. They may exhibit intolerance to everyday frustrations, or exaggerate them or catastrophize. They may be pessimistic. For example:

'Nothing ever works out right!'
'This is all your fault!'
'These things never happen to me!'
'I don't know why I bother. Life sucks.'

Entrenched patterns of behaviour

People who are either not aware of or avoid uncomfortable feelings in themselves may end up repeating the same old behaviour time and time again because they do not stop to reflect on their feelings, thoughts and actions.

Suppressing thoughts and feelings can be dangerous. A lack of insight means an individual may act in the same way repeatedly in difficult situations. When their words and deeds meet rejection it serves to reinforce their reliance on passive aggressive ways of dealing with unwanted feelings; hence it becomes a vicious pattern that can prevent the person gaining emotional sustenance and support from other people.

Emotional disconnection

People who exhibit passive aggressiveness often mistake using polite and cooperative words as the same as building good rapport with others. So they may well, at least on the surface, agree to do things even when they do not want to. Emotional disconnection means that their agreement to cooperate becomes an act of hostile cooperation.

'Yes, I'll do that for you tomorrow.'
'Yup, whatever.'
'Whatever pleases you.'
'Yes, yes. I heard you. No need to keep going on.'
'I said I would do it, so stop going on.'
'Yes, all right (*sighing*). I'll do it when I can.'

Their real thoughts and opinions are not expressed, however, and may gnaw at them and cause resentment. The more they agree to things they do not want to do, the more resentment builds up, which aggravates their passive aggressive tendencies. This incongruence between what they say and what they genuinely feel and think creates a barrier to effective communication and ultimately to relations with other people.

Dispirited behaviour

People who display passive aggressive tendencies often look to their partner to tell them what to do, even though they resent it. Because they tend to resent change, they often find it difficult to accept changes in arrangements and routines. This can lead to them 'digging their heels in' and becoming even more dispirited and uncooperative.

Ways to counter passive aggression when communicating with other people

Refuse to engage with passive aggression In order to avoid passive aggression, we first need to recognize the style of communication and common behaviours of the passive aggressive. Engage in good self-talk and make a commitment that when we hear it or see it in ourselves or other people we will not entertain or tolerate it in any way.

Don't overreact People with passive aggressive tendencies do what they do because of them; often it has little to do with us. Taking this broader perspective can reduce the possibility of misunderstanding, lessen the impact of the hurts they dish out and helps us see that this is a problem behaviour for the other person to overcome.

Avoid encouraging passive aggression in others In relationships it is important to avoid behaving and communicating in ways that may trigger the individual's worst passive aggressive instincts. For instance, you may unwittingly indulge your partner's passive aggression because you don't communicate with him or her in an assertive way or set firm boundaries. Or unwittingly over the years you may become your partner's caretaker, always cleaning up after him or her, undoing the damage done, or rescuing him or her from every crisis.

Conversely you may be overly critical, berating the person for not taking responsibility, or setting expectations to which you know the person is likely not to respond. By being overly critical, you may take on the role of the critical parent or authority figure that sets off this behaviour in the first place and unwittingly encourage your partner to re-engage with the past and exacerbate passive aggressive tendencies. Your relationship can end up as a constant power struggle. Some people try to change chronically passive aggressive individuals through endless discussion about their behaviour. Such efforts often end in frustration. Passive aggressive people change only when they become more self-aware. The best way to deal with people with passive aggressive tendencies is by taking charge of your own.

Amplify unreasonable behaviour In confrontational situations where people with passive aggressive tendencies are on the defensive, they may project unwanted feelings and issues on to you, or some other person, or family pet, or even an inanimate object. In such circumstances, pointing out the 'elephant in the room' sometimes can have a positive effect as their unreasonable behaviour is reflected back. Try to avoid accusations and statements that begin with 'you', which are more likely to trigger defensiveness. For example:

> 'It seems to me that you're angry at me for asking this of you.'
> 'It is unacceptable to kick the dog. He isn't the cause of the upset.'
> 'I won't tolerate this attack. It's unwarranted.'

Bringing the anger into the open can draw other people's attention to someone's unreasonable behaviour and if the discussion is getting heated or potentially threatening, it may help alert bystanders to the situation and predicament that you are in.

Back away from further discussion Don't argue with the person's denial of hostility. Regardless of what he or she continues to say or deny, make clear what you're willing to do to sort things out. Using sentences that begin with 'I', 'we' and 'let's' shows that you are willing to share responsibility for working things out. For that reason, it is best to avoid making accusatory comments or using sentences that start with 'you', as these could make the individual even more defensive.

> 'Let's see if we can find some way to resolve this.'
> 'I find this upsetting, can't we resolve it some other way?'
> 'Let's wait until we're both in the frame of mind to sort this problem out in a way that works for both of us.'

Sometimes, however, despite all your good intentions, things escalate and there may come a time when the best thing to do is calmly back away from further discussion, leaving the person who is passive aggressive with the knowledge that the anger is affecting his or her behaviour. By calmly but assertively sharing your awareness of his or her passive aggression, you will send a powerful message that the behaviour cannot continue.

'Before this gets out of hand, I am going to stop this conversation.'
'You seem very angry right now and I find your remarks offensive, so I am going to end this discussion now.'
'I don't think your anger towards me is warranted and I don't like the hostile way you are talking to me. So I am going to end the conversation and walk away now.'

Ways to avoid passive aggression ourselves

Accept that anger is not a bad thing to feel or express Anger is a normal and natural feeling and it is acceptable to express it. The biggest obstacle to assertive communication is the belief that anger is bad and expressing it is inappropriate.

Be assertive Instead of requesting help and support in roundabout ways, as those who are passive aggressive tend to do, find ways to make assertive requests in a straightforward fashion. A passive aggressive request might go like this (loaded with sarcasm and put-downs): 'I've got such a busy day ahead full of important meetings. After doing whatever it is you do all day, would you mind taking this parcel to the post office for me? If you're not too busy, of course.' An assertive request is a straightforward one such as: 'If you have time today, would you mind taking this parcel to the post office for me?'

Acknowledge other people's perspectives and feelings Showing that you can appreciate other people's perspectives and acknowledge their feelings helps to foster more respectful communication. This doesn't mean agreeing or approving; rather, it is an act of validation. It is the recognition and acceptance of other people's thoughts, feelings and behaviours. Someone with passive aggressive tendencies may be used to feeling rejected, ignored or judged. Invalidation is emotionally upsetting for anyone and disrupts relationships and creates emotional distance.

Maintain respectful communication Being assertive in your communication means collaborating too in order to achieve a situation where both people are able to assert their points of view but

also compromise, when necessary. Maintaining a respectful attitude, keeping eye contact and managing your own emotions and
thoughts will help you maintain the 'I'm OK, you're OK' position
(see Table 2, p. 43, and the portion from it given in Table 3, below)
in our communications with others and may persuade them to
steer towards that position, too.

Recognizing that your needs matter as much as anyone else's may
involve compromise, but it also means standing up for yourself and
finding ways to express your point clearly and confidently. Being
an assertive communicator enhances relationships as other people
know where they stand and it helps build your self-esteem.

The next chapter discusses covert aggression and how to spot and
deal with it. It is a particularly pernicious form of aggression and
involves tactics of deceit and manipulation.

Table 3 'I'm OK, you're OK': belief

I'm OK, you're OK
Belief
I believe and act as if we both deserve respect. We are equally entitled to have things done our way

6

Bringing covert aggression into the open

People who engage in acts of covert aggression do their best to keep their aggressive intentions and behaviours hidden. They are devious and underhand in the ways they exploit others. Here's a case in point.

Paul, an office worker, speaks honestly and openly to his manager, Susan, about the unequal way work seems to be allocated by the manager among the team. Susan, who is a domineering character, responds by saying that she constantly feels as if unreasonable demands are being placed on her by her team, especially Paul, who she says is out to cause trouble for her even though she treats him well (casting herself as the 'victim'). She insists that she works hard to allocate work fairly, but that no one seems to appreciate it. She tells anyone who will listen that Paul is always complaining (guilt-tripping) and criticizing her unfairly. She wonders (out loud) why he continues to work there if it makes him so miserable. The rest of the team, she says, get on with things without moaning, so why should she pay attention to him and his incessant complaining? Susan hopes this veiled threat will manipulate Paul into keeping quiet, but it does not. Instead, he sees what she is trying to do and is aggravated by her antics. He lets other people know how she has responded to his complaint and how indignant he feels, hoping that they will come out in support of him, since he knows other people have been complaining among themselves about the heavy and uneven distribution of work in recent months. His colleagues, however, perhaps out of fear of comeback, refuse to get involved and back away from the situation. This leaves Paul thinking that he must be an unjust attacker. So he relents and puts up with the situation, despite his efforts to address things and see changes at work. Things end up more difficult than ever and he feels powerless to do anything about it other than look for a new job.

This situation highlights a number of issues about covert aggression and those who engage in it. Covert aggression is at the heart of most interpersonal manipulation. Someone skilled in the tactics of covert aggression will attempt to make you doubt yourself, explain yourself, question your judgement and, if they can, they will get you to back down or surrender to their view and control. It is targeted hostility. Covert aggressors use subtle tactics to blind you to their self-serving agendas and attempts to exert control over you.

Recognizing common manipulation tactics

Manipulating bystanders

So often in situations of covert aggression and abuse, the victim is left without help. So why don't people help when they witness others in compromised and dangerous situations? In Chapter 2, the bystander effect was discussed and the human propensity to be passive in the face of threatening situations happening to someone else. It is known, for instance, that the greater the number of bystanders, the less likely it is that any one of them will help. Researchers have studied the phenomenon and attribute the occurrence of passive bystanding to a 'diffusion of responsibility': when people believe there are other witnesses to an emergency, they feel less personal responsibility to intervene. They assume that someone else will help.

While passivity can be simply the first reaction to perceived danger and an avoidance strategy employed in the hope that the problem will go away, in some people it can indicate something more sinister. Individuals who harbour feelings of envy, or disgust, or who view the targeted individual as somehow different from them, an outsider, not someone in the 'in-group', may passively or actively connive in the hostilities they witness. The reasons people join forces with aggressors are manifold: they may fear punishment if they stand up to the aggressor, they themselves may bear a grudge towards the targeted person or group, or they may feel no connection with the target and shut off from feeling concern because of this. And some individuals may take pleasure in seeing someone other than themselves getting hurt. Sadly, as previously discussed, sadism is more common – an everyday phenomenon – than is openly acknowledged.

People who engage in covert aggression as a way of exerting control over other people usually have amassed an arsenal of interpersonal tactics to effectively manipulate and control those around them. Bystander passivity and other influences on human behaviour can discourage a lot of us from helping one another in times of danger and distress.

Covert aggressors manipulate anyone and everyone they can. They take advantage of people's passivity and fear and silence about abuses and violence that bystanders witness. The covert aggressor will usually identify a specific target, perhaps someone who is assertive enough to speak out or is prepared to challenge the status quo, as Paul did in the example at the beginning of this chapter. People like Paul threaten the covert aggressor's power and control in his or her sphere of influence, whether that is the workplace, social circle or domestic setting. It is common to see covert aggressors at work employing these manipulation tactics online, especially nowadays with the increasing reliance on social media, as a means to gain influence and social prestige.

Impression management

It is usual for people to want to present themselves in ways that aid and enhance their social influence. Shakespeare crafted the famous line, 'All the world's a stage, and all the men and women merely players' (*As You Like It*, Act II, Scene VII), highlighting the way individuals project a desired image of themselves on an audience for self-serving reasons. Impression management is a process in which people attempt to influence the perceptions of others about a person, situation or event. While it is not behaviour unique to aggressors, as we all engage in impression-managing situations to some extent, it is synonymous with self-presentation. A lot of covert aggressors are fixated with power and control. Those who have narcissistic or sociopathic traits may attempt to steady an unstable sense of self-image by impression managing and/or staging events.

Impression management involves people attempting to influence the perception of their image by using strategies to shape the social identity they project to others. It is a mainstay tactic of online covert aggressors who may adopt any number of self-presentation strategies, such as the ones in the following list.

- **Self-disclosing** Individuals may self-disclose – that is, identify what makes them 'them' – to others in an attempt to make them find the individual's personality attractive or believe that they have a lot in common.
- **Boasting** This has to be tempered with false modesty, enough to gain acceptance and to be liked by others.
- **Flattery or praise** This increases social attractiveness. It is useful for swelling the number of people willing to passively overlook or actively support an attack on a specific individual or group at some later stage.
- **Ingratiation** This involves managing appearances and trying to fit in, aligning actions and making actions seem appealing or understandable and imposing roles/identities on other people. Aggressive humour can be used to ingratiate the 'in-group', together with sarcasm and belittling of those who are not in the 'in-group'. This serves to encourage followers to engage in and be compliant with any aggressive behaviour later shown towards the intended target group or individual.
- **Alter casting** This involves imposing identities on other people. Alter casting is usually carried out as a way of forcing people to accept certain roles. Covert aggressors may adopt the victim role or blame the victim; blaming is a way of avoiding culpability. For example: 'I know that if he harassed you and complained about you all the time, you wouldn't tolerate it either . . .' (to persuade bystanders to view the person that the covert aggressor has targeted as a troublemaker) or, 'You're someone with integrity. I've seen your upset reaction when your colleague always has a go at me. I'm glad that some people see the bullying going on around here.' This tactic is often used when the covert aggressor adopts the role of the victim, as in the example at the start of the chapter. It is a means of getting bystanders to become involved in the targeting and abuse of the real victim.

Internet-based communication tools provide new opportunities for impression management, especially via social networking sites. Many of us select carefully chosen images of our physical appearance and are specific in how we present our interests, our careers, talents and competence. We do so largely for social approval from others. Behind much of this self-promotion and self-presentation is a desire to stave off rejection and criticism from social groups.

In social networking sites, users can create custom profile pages and fill them with information of their choosing about themselves. Social network users can employ protective measures for image management. For instance, users can 'untag' an undesirable photo on social media sites or request the photo is removed. Other strategies can be used when a 'friend' posts an undesirable comment about the user. Maintaining one's self-esteem is an important motivation for self-image management online.

In Chapter 2 I highlighted several common strategies of online aggressors identified by Dr Claire Hardaker, who studies the language of aggression. The online strategies she identified include 'digression', which involves straying from the purpose of the discussion or forum and introducing entirely irrelevant topics; criticizing others excessively for an offence of which the critic is also guilty (termed 'hypo-criticizing'); 'antipathizing', where the person engaging in online aggression proactively and usually covertly exploits a sensitive discussion by being deliberately controversial or provocative. Other strategies involve 'endangering', where the covert aggressor masquerades as a help or advice giver while actually causing harm to another user.

For example, a previously unknown person leaves a comment on a Facebook public page, which has a focus on the topic of recovery from abuse:

Hi. I am suffering quite a lot. I am reaching out online to the chronically ill and to abuse survivors. I am still being stalked, bullied and manipulated through profiles. It is causing me a lot of stress and anxiety. What do you recommend that I do, as this is having a severe impact on my quality of life? As you know, my background is counselling and health care, so I've had the skills for many years before specializing in victims of abuses, and survivors in particular. It's good to support others, especially when isolated within society.

We previously discussed a meet-up in a coffee shop or somewhere close to your house, since you know I know the area well. It will be a family trip. I think it will be later than I thought, though, and near Christmas when we can get to you.

This is an attempt at impression management. This individual was not known to the page facilitators at all. The woman issues a veiled threat by implying that she knows where the person lives. Most concerning of all, she employs endangering tactics. She is masquerading as a benevolent person, out to help survivors of abuse and setting up an online recovery group for the purpose. In fact, some weeks later her mal-intent was exposed when it came to light that she had intimidated and harassed multiple individuals, including many who were survivors of abuse, whom she had invited to join her online recovery group.

Gaslighting

As mentioned in Chapter 2, gaslighting is a form of psychological abuse in which false information is presented in such a way as to make the target doubt their own memory and perception. The person who is gaslighted no longer trusts their own perception of the situation. The process distorts their sense of reality and makes them disbelieve what they see. Anyone can become the victim of another person's gaslighting moves and it can take place in any kind of relationship.

Gaslighting is a form of mental abuse. Instances may range simply from the denial by a covert abuser that previous abusive incidents ever occurred, up to the staging of bizarre events with the intention of disorientating the targeted person. Here are some examples of this type of abuse.

Refusing to listen to the targeted person's perspective

'I'm not listening to you going on about that again. You're crazy!'
'You're just trying to confuse me.'

Calling into question another person's memory or perception of events

Intentionally questioning the individual's perception of events makes them doubt their own motivations and perceptions.

'You always get the facts wrong.'
'You said that before and you were wrong.'
'I wouldn't trust you to remember. You've such a poor memory.'
'You always get the wrong end of the stick.'
'That's not what happened at all!'
'It wasn't like that. You always distort things. John saw what happened as well and his recollection of events is the same as mine.'

Discounting

The abuser will start to question the experiences, thoughts and opinions with frequent put-downs.

'You see everything in a negative way.'
'You are overly sensitive.'
'You always exaggerate.'
'You are such a drama queen.'
'Well, you obviously never trusted me.'
'You have an overactive imagination.'

Diverting

This is where the covert abuser interrupts and gains the upper hand and control of the conversation by questioning the motives of the other person.

'I'm not going to listen to all that crazy stuff again.'
'Where did you get an absurd idea like that?'
'Your thinking is very disturbed, do you know that?'
'You deliberately set out to hurt me by going on like this.'

Minimizing

Sometimes the person using covert aggressive tactics pretends to forget things that have really occurred or significantly plays them down.

'You're going to let something like that come between us?'
'What are you talking about?'
'You're making that up.'

How to deal effectively with covert aggressors

Trust and act on your instincts

Sometimes we are prompted to respond to certain people and situations by instinct. Most instincts are accompanied by some kind of physical sensation, from goose bumps to a tightening in the chest. A research study from 2012 showed that forced to choose between two options based on instinct alone, participants made the right call up to 90 per cent of the time, indicating that intuition is a surprisingly powerful and accurate tool.[1] However, some people are more 'instinct alert' than others, while some people are, or become over time, what is termed 'instinct injured'. Injury to our instinctive survival apparatus can occur through trauma, illness or other factors. In such circumstances the individual is unable to recognize, or process and decode these instincts that alert the body to danger. Those who are instinct injured are more inclined to be risk-averse and apathetic to their own and others' plight in times of danger. Being reliant only on the rational mind can lead an individual to overthink, overanalyse and make poorer decisions than if they follow their intuition and do what *feels* right. We are 'feeling creatures that think', insists American neuroanatomist Jill Bolte Taylor (quoted in Chapter 3). We need to be alert to instincts to help us react quickly in times of danger.

To hone intuition, the brain needs more emotional information to work with. Engaging in the art of self-reflection may lead to greater self-awareness and, with that, we may become more alert to 'self' and the sensations that affect us, as well as more alert to ourselves and how we interact with our surroundings. Becoming more aware of yourself and the world around you involves awareness of your inner workings – your feelings, emotions, values, beliefs, strengths and weaknesses – as well as awareness of how you communicate with the people in your life and all the ways in which you manage your interpersonal relationships.

Some people practise mindfulness as a means of improving their awareness of self and maintaining a moment-by-moment awareness of thoughts, feelings, bodily sensations and surrounding environment. Mindfulness also involves acceptance, meaning that we pay attention to our thoughts and feelings without judging them as 'right' or 'wrong' ways to think or feel in a given moment. When we practise mindfulness, our thoughts tune into what we're sensing in the present moment. There is some evidence to suggest that regularly engaging in mindfulness exercises can reduce anger, hostility and mood disturbances and reduce symptoms of stress. Here are a few key things that you need to do when practising mindfulness.

- Pay close attention to your breathing, especially when you are feeling intense emotions.

- Notice what you're sensing in a given moment – the sights, sounds and smells that ordinarily you are not conscious of.
- Recognize that your thoughts and emotions are passing and do not define you.
- Tune into your body's physical sensations, from the water hitting your skin in the shower to the way your body rests in your office chair.

Bring hostility into the open

Covert aggressors get away with their behaviour most often because their abuses are hidden from public view and attention. This means that the targeted person is left unsupported by those who would be likely to help if they saw the bigger picture and the aggressor's behaviour for what it is. It has to be made apparent for all to see. One way we can do this is to refuse to engage in one-on-one conversations with the covert aggressor. Ask for a third party to be present when at all possible so that any hostility can be witnessed. The other important task is to stay calm and act reasonably while amplifying the other person's unreasonableness and hostility. For example:

> 'Calling me offensive names isn't acceptable.'
> 'So you think it is OK to threaten me?'
> 'So you think it is OK to hit out at me?'
> 'Do you think it's acceptable to intimidate me by shouting like that?

Communicate assertively

Communicating assertively means clearly and calmly expressing what you want without being either too passive or too aggressive. Boundaries are needed. Tips for communicating assertively include being clear and direct:

> 'I am going to end this conversation now.'
> 'I find that unacceptable and I won't tolerate it.'

Describe how another person's behaviour makes you feel so that the person is aware of the consequences of their actions.

> 'Your shouting scares me . . . please lower your voice.'

Refuse to collude with other people's abuses

People who turn a blind eye – or worse, go along with and collude with the covert abuser's perspective of the situation – are an integral part of the covert abuser's arsenal. Covert abusers often have an uncanny knack of knowing who will assist them in bringing down their target. Many people in everyday life can find themselves an accomplice or acting indifferently or with cowardice in fearful situations.

Otherwise fair-minded people can become involved in abusive situations, wittingly or unwittingly. This may be a consequence of poor judgement or it may be linked to reduced empathy for the targeted person. The passive bystander might bear a grudge, be jealous, angry, or have a sense of being let down by the targeted person and as a consequence want to see the individual defeated. Other times it is because they do not want to see 'bad' in others so they choose not to do so. Or they might not possess the moral courage to help another person.

It is in this situation that people blindly follow leaders motivated only by self-interest. As mentioned in Chapter 2, this sort of behaviour was demonstrated in experiments by Professor Stanley Milgram in the 1960s, who set up an experiment to test the human propensity to obey orders. In the experiment, a 'teacher' was told to deliver electric shocks to a 'learner' when they got the answer to a question wrong. The 'teacher' subject believed that for each wrong answer, the 'learner' was receiving actual shocks (in truth there were no shocks). Milgram's experiments, and others like it repeated since, show that a person of authority can strongly influence other people's behaviour, with appalling consequences.

Both empathic concern and indifference towards others are contagious behaviours – they spread from one person to another. Consequently, one person who acts with empathy or apathy potentially has the power to infect or influence everyone around them. Breaking from the apathy around us and responding empathically is a step towards building a culture of cooperation. We each can make a difference, for individually as well as collectively we make up the culture we live in. So, if you are harmed by a covert aggressor or you have witnessed someone else being abused, and if you or another person has been or remains in danger, you need to think about your obligation to report what you have witnessed to the police and other relevant agencies. By coming forward and reporting what you experienced or witnessed you may prevent the same problem happening again to someone else. Evidence from victims and witnesses is important because it demonstrates the distress and damage of covert aggressive behaviour in our communities. Apathy equates to collusion; hence turning a blind eye is not an option for a person of integrity.

Legislation

Individuals who control other people by covert means – in daily life, via social media or by spying on them online – can face up to five years in prison under a law that came into force in England and Wales in December 2015. The legislation targets those who subject spouses, partners and family members to psychological and emotional torment, but stop short of violence. It paves the way for charges in cases where there is evidence of repeated 'controlling or coercive behaviour'. The type of abuse covered by the new offence includes a pattern of threats, humiliation and intimidation. They may involve stopping someone from socializing, controlling their social media accounts, surveillance through apps and dictating what individuals wear and spend. This sort of controlling or coercive behaviour limits an individual's basic human rights, such as freedom of movement and independence, and can be very harmful in relationships where one person holds more power than the other. The new offence criminalizes patterns of such behaviour against an intimate partner or family member. Critical to the offence is the repeated or continuous nature of the conduct and the ability of a reasonable person to appreciate that the behaviour will have a serious effect on its victim. Evidence could include emails and bank records, so it is important to document events and keep safe evidence of this kind.

Covert aggression and harassment in the workplace should not be tolerated. Sexual harassment is one of the most common forms of covert harassment and in the UK it is specifically outlawed by the Equality Act 2010. The Advisory, Conciliation and Arbitration Service (ACAS), an organization devoted to preventing and resolving employment disputes, argues that it is in the interest of the organization you work for to make it clear what sorts of behaviour would be considered harassment and what would constitute bullying. Bullying is most often characterized as offensive, intimidating, malicious or insulting behaviour, and an abuse or misuse of power through means that undermine, humiliate, denigrate or injure the recipient. Harassment is unwanted conduct related to a relevant protected characteristic, which has the purpose or effect of violating an individual's dignity or creating an intimidating, hostile, degrading, humiliating or offensive environment for that individual.

It is good practice for employers to give examples of what is unacceptable behaviour in their organization, which may include: spreading malicious rumours; insulting someone (particularly on the grounds of age, race, sex, disability, sexual orientation and religion or belief); copying documents that are critical about someone to others who do not need to know; ridiculing or demeaning someone (picking on them or setting them up to fail); exclusion or victimization, unfair treatment, overbearing supervision or other misuse of power or position; unwelcome sexual advances (touching, standing too close, displaying offensive materials, asking for sexual favours, making decisions on the basis of sexual advances being accepted or rejected); making threats or comments about job security without foundation; deliberately undermining a competent worker by overloading and constant criticism; preventing individuals progressing by intentionally blocking promotion or training opportunities.

If the covert aggressor is a friend or neighbour, be vigilant and record any unusual goings-on. If you are experiencing intimidating behaviour or harassment, do not ignore it – most of the time it is unlikely to go away without some kind of action. Do not feel that it is your fault, or fear being labelled as a troublemaker for bringing it to the attention of others and the police. People who are involved in harassing behaviour often display it as a form of control and 'superiority' over you, so ignoring it could be seen as a sign of success by the covert aggressor harassing you.

Even if you have only been harassed once, do not ever hesitate to contact someone for more help. If the situation warrants it – for instance, if your safety or someone else's is at risk, or there has been damage done to property – inform your local police and ask for help. Ask them about the Protection from Harassment Act of 1997

(PFHA) and other possible legal avenues that could be open to you. The PFHA defines harassment as a 'course of conduct' amounting to harassment that must involve conduct on at least two occasions. Originally these occasions needed to involve the same person, but in 2005 the Act was amended by the Serious Organised Crime and Police Act so that 'pursuing a course of conduct' could mean approaching two people just once. Ask the police if they are able to take action on your behalf under relevant legislation and in particular the PFHA.

If in doubt about going to the police, you could talk to a harassment adviser (you may have one in your workplace or organization) or seek the help of a counsellor. Do not ever approach the neighbour or person who is harassing you if you are in any way worried that there may be actual physical danger or threatened violence. Call the police at once if this is the case. If you decide to approach the person responsible for causing you harassment, think seriously about your actions and take due care over your safety. Do NOT go alone; take a friend or relative with you. By taking a witness it could be useful to have a third-party account of what was said and done; the harasser then cannot claim that you did not ask them to stop their harassing behaviour. Above all, your safety is paramount; do NOT place yourself in unnecessary danger.

7

Dealing with overt aggression

Violence and aggression are major public health problems worldwide. Each year, millions of people die as the result of injuries due to violence.

Substance use sometimes plays a role in violence and hostility; users of alcohol, steroids and stimulant drugs such as cocaine and amphetamines may have greater propensity for hostility and aggression. Aggressive behaviours can also be exhibited by people who are physically unwell. Aggression can stem from genetic predisposition, other biological origins and mental health concerns. Aggression is a common symptom among patients with dementia. Hitting, kicking, biting and pushing are associated with cognitive decline. Brain lesions that affect frontal lobe function, including tumours and traumatic injuries, are associated with disinhibition, aggression and violence.

There is also evidence linking violent episodes to disorders associated with a lack of empathy or concern for others such as antisocial personality disorder (ASPD). Furthermore, individuals with high levels of hostility and low levels of insight are at greater risk for violent offending. Frequent aggression can result in time in prison, financial problems because of legal fees, relationship problems and disruption to an individual's physical and emotional well-being. Physical aggression in an intimate relationship can increase the risk of separation or divorce and children caught up in such hostile conditions at home can be negatively affected by both verbal and physical aggression.

We may not be able to prevent violence occurring in everyday life, but we can help ourselves in the face of attack. This chapter discusses what we can do to help ourselves when on the receiving end of aggression or threatened with violence, online and in daily life, and highlights how we can keep our own aggression in check.

Overt aggression linked to frustration-anger

Although in some populations aggression is a common way of acting, individual differences in overt aggressive behaviour are seen emerging in early childhood. Aggression is strongly associated with problems in social relationships and functioning. The emergence and persistence of high levels of overt aggressive behaviour in early childhood is one of the strongest and most consistent predictors of antisocial behavioural disorders in later life. Decades of theory and research have established a body of evidence suggesting that children who show high levels of frustration-anger become more overtly aggressive as adults. The link between frustration-anger and overt aggression is that those children and adults who become frustrated and angry are more likely to lash out at others.

When you are open, direct and obvious in your manner of fighting, your behaviour is best described as overtly aggressive. The following definitions apply to overt aggression:

- **impulsivity** a behavioural state characterized by diminished restraint to action in response to some stimulus;
- **agitation** a state of emotional arousal or restlessness;
- **aggression** physical violence towards people or objects or verbal threats and intimidation;
- **violence** overt physical aggression that has the potential consequence of physical harm to another person or object.

Aggression is either viewed as natural and largely self-defence or a way of combating social injustice, or it is viewed as pathological, when an individual's inner nature has become twisted and their outward behaviour is antisocial. The latter kind is sometimes called 'predatory aggression' and is a purposeful, premeditated type of aggression that can be physical, emotional or both. People who engage in predatory aggression may act without provocation in order to gain a particular outcome. This form of aggression includes deliberate and callous behaviours often carried out by people who feel no remorse for their actions. It can include verbal aggression such as spreading gossip, attempts at tarnishing someone's reputation, social exclusion, or otherwise hurting someone.

In Chapter 1, I described two cases, the first involving a cyclist and a car driver. The driver swears at the cyclist out of the window then gets out, shouting a tirade of abuse at the cyclist, who he accuses of damaging his car. After this verbal outburst, he threatens to kill the cyclist. In the second, also real-life case, a man was jailed for two years after he attacked a neighbour, punching him in the eye, apparently for no reason other than being told to calm down.

Some behaviours antagonize those who are easily frustrated, as these two examples illustrate. These can include humiliating or talking down to someone, telling individuals they are wrong to feel or behave as they do and trivializing a person's problems or concerns. Be aware of your own reactions to aggression from other people and try to remain calm. If you respond aggressively, you will reinforce the other person's behaviour. Try also to defuse the aggression as early as possible by showing empathy. It is best to avoid aggression rather than try to calm things down when aggression has started to escalate. So, keep a non-threatening stance and avoid appearing confrontational by keeping physical movements calm. Also respect personal space – yours and theirs. Encourage the individual to take responsibility for their own behaviour and at the same time avoid any expression of power, for example by saying, 'You must stop behaving like this', or 'You must calm down'. Do be alert to signs of aggression, such as the ones listed below.

- **Appearance** Is the person intoxicated? Does the person have an unusual appearance, such as being bloodstained or dishevelled? Does he or she have a weapon?
- **Posture** Is the person restless or agitated in some way? Are his or her fists clenched? Does the person invade your personal space? Does he or she have a hostile expression?
- **Speech** Is the person abusive or threatening? Is his or her voice raised?

How to deal with escalating aggression

The following are some guidelines on how to deal with an aggressive situation.

If you interrupt the aggressor when they are speaking or shouting, do so in a calm but assured manner. Do not turn your back on the person or walk in front of them or encroach on their personal space. Keep far enough away to be out of striking distance.

Plan your escape route and theirs, too. Unless the violence is premeditated (as in predatory aggression) then usually the person would rather escape the situation than attack you. Therefore, if you have the means to back away then do, or else try to give the aggressor the means by which to escape from the confrontation. An exit or escape route open to the aggressor may prevent them from feeling out of control or threatened – situations that may escalate their aggression levels.

Safety is paramount at all times, so exiting an escalating aggression situation can be the brave and right thing to do. Do not try to deal with a violent person by yourself when the violence has escalated; always seek help when possible. Do not attempt to disarm a person with a weapon. If the person claims to have a concealed weapon or you suspect they do, leave the situation if you can and as soon as possible, then call the police.

If you cannot escape the situation, here are some suggested courses of action.

- Be prepared to protect yourself from harm.
- Avoid arguing and keep the individual talking as a means of preventing the person acting violently.
- If the person becomes calmer, suggest that he or she put the weapon down. If the weapon is put down, leave it in sight, but do not take it (best to wait until help arrives). If help has not been summoned and the person has downed arms, then talk as much as necessary to defuse the situation.
- Make use of whatever surrounds you to act as a shield if violence occurs.
- Escape when opportunity presents itself.

Restraining the aggressive impulse

In severe cases of impulsive aggression, especially if it results in physical aggression, it is important that individuals take responsibility and seek support. Support may involve cognitive behavioural therapy (CBT). CBT teaches individuals how to manage aversive stimuli in the day-to-day environment and may prevent aggressive impulses that can trigger explosive outbursts. Specific techniques used in CBT include:

- **cognitive restructuring** modifying faulty assumptions and dysfunctional thoughts about frustrating situations and perceived threats;
- **relaxation training** deep breathing and muscle relaxation exercises while imagining situations that provoke anger;
- **coping skills training** role-playing potentially provocative situations and rehearsing responses, such as walking away.

In mild cases, the more you understand your anger and what stimulates it, the more likely it is that you will acquire ways to manage it better and stop it becoming aggressive. This may involve you accepting that your feelings are neither good nor bad, but that they are trying to convey something to you. When you feel angry or experience any feelings related to anger (upset, annoyance, frustration, resentment or feeling judgemental), then undertake some self-reflection and ask yourself questions such as, 'Is my anger masking some other feelings?' If the answer is 'yes', then acknowledge these feelings.

Here are some means by which to manage symptoms of frustration and anger when they surface in order to diminish your tendency to be aggressive.

Moods

You may be someone who experiences mood swings – low moods, bad moods, increased anxiety or irritability. You may occasionally overreact to things that normally wouldn't bother you. This is normal. Try to find new ways of coping with emotions such as anger, upset, annoyance, stress. Sometimes just allowing yourself time out in the day to recognize how you are feeling can help. One can permit feelings and accept them as neither good nor bad but indicators of our well-being, without always having to act on them. One way to become more conversant with how we feel is to take some quiet time out of the day and press the 'pause' button. This buys some time out from your anger and frustration. You might want to ask yourself these questions.

- What will I do to press the pause button? (Walk away, count to ten, distract yourself, keep quiet, bite your tongue.)
- What things might I try to stop me getting angry? (Breathing, self-talk, exercise, talking to someone I trust, assertiveness.)

It can be difficult to identify your thoughts, so another way of looking at the issue is to view thoughts as 'self-talk', or talking things over in your head. This is a normal thing to do and it can be really helpful. You can use self-talk to help when you are going into a difficult situation in which you may possibly get angry. You can also use it to get through the situation, or to review afterwards what you did in the situation.

Frustration

People with anger difficulties often talk about first being frustrated and, after that sets in, getting angry. Frustration is a feeling that we all experience from time to time, especially when we are thwarted or hindered while trying to do something specific or reach a goal. It is what you feel when you expect something different from what really happened. On the plus side, frustration can be helpful as it leads to new ways of thinking about a problem. Frustration is basically about not getting what we want, or getting what we do not want. Finding ways to manage frustration may improve our sense of well-being in everyday life.

A variety of factors can trigger frustration. These include:

- thoughts – unrealistic expectations, plans, ideas for self or others (thoughts that include the words 'should', 'must' and 'ought': 'You should do what I tell you');
- bodily sensations – muscles tensing;
- situations – particular places or tasks;
- relationships – particular people.

Frustration often occurs when we have expectations for ourselves or others that are too high or unattainable. We may have to alter our perspective or way of thinking. We may need to become what is called 'frustration tolerant'. To be frustration tolerant is to continue living a balanced, healthy life despite encountering repeated interferences and obstacles. Frustration tolerance refers to how robust we are in the face of life's stressors and challenges. Low frustration tolerance happens when a person gets easily frustrated when they cannot get what they want. Their frustration is intolerable and they cannot cope. This way of thinking leads to the discomfort being increased. People with low frustration tolerance underestimate their ability to cope with the discomfort ('I can't bear it!' or

'I can't stand it'). Describing something as 'intolerable' frequently makes situations appear more daunting or off-putting than they actually are.

The most effective approach to overcoming a low tolerance of frustration is to develop an alternative and positive attitude to high tolerance of it. High frustration tolerance is the ability to tolerate discomfort while waiting to get what you want. Basically it is about toughing things out. Increasing tolerance for frustration helps us to experience normal levels of healthy annoyance in response to being blocked. High frustration tolerance enables us to be more effective at solving problems or accepting things that, at least at present, cannot be changed.

Examples of high frustration tolerance statements are:

'This is an uncomfortable situation, but I can stand the discomfort.'
'This situation is hard to bear, but I can bear it – some difficult things are worth tolerating.'
'Even if I feel like I can't take it any more, past experience has shown that I probably can.'

To increase tolerance for frustration, ask these types of questions.

'Can I remember being in this situation before and coping with it?'
'Is it true that I can't stand this situation or is it just that I don't like this situation?'
'Is this situation truly unbearable or is it really just very difficult to bear?'

Being less extreme in our judgement of negative situations can help us have less extreme emotional responses, such as energy-depleting anger. Many situations are difficult to tolerate, but we need to remember at such times that we have tolerated similar in the past.

The best approach might be to find ways of controlling the degree of frustration that we experience in daily life. This may be achieved by changing the things we do, or thoughts we have, when we feel frustrated. Alternatively, there may be nothing we can do – in which case, it may be less energy consuming if we are able to learn to accept and tolerate the uncomfortable experiences.

Venting

Venting means letting out pent-up feelings of anger or getting things off your chest. Venting is often explosive and can be very aggressive. When we vent our anger, we often feel better immediately afterwards. However, not long after the venting most people report feeling guilty, ashamed or sad for the hurt they have caused to the other person. Originally venting was thought to be healthy for reducing anger difficulties. However, the sway of recent evidence suggests that venting is not as helpful as once supposed because it increases the chances of further anger in the future.

Reduce venting by taking the following steps, which may help you to express your anger in a healthier way.

- Recognize and label your angry feelings.
- 'I am feeling angry because . . .'
- Is it important or unimportant?
- If it is important, can you influence or control it?
- If it is important and you can control it, are there strategies that are necessary in order to implement the actions? If so, then list them. If the incident is not important, dismiss it and move on to other issues.

Anger rumination

Anger rumination can focus on injustice, angry memories, thoughts of revenge and angry afterthoughts. In ruminative anger, the body's cortisol and adrenaline levels increase as part of the body's fight or flight system. However, if we do not fight or run, the cortisol and adrenaline stay in the body, affecting the immune system, sleep and emotional well-being. These hormones have been linked with both heart disease and depression.

The way we think about things affects our emotions and bodies. If, for example, you are hungry and see your favourite meal, your mouth will water, but just thinking or imagining your favourite meal will have a similar effect because our thoughts stimulate areas of the brain responsible for digestion. Likewise, ruminating about something will trigger the fight or flight response and get our bodies psyched up.

As with all aspects of anger, the first task is to recognize when we are doing it. So whenever you start to dwell on something that makes you feel angry, remind yourself that you are ruminating – 'Warning! I'm ruminating!' – and stop as quickly as possible. However, this may be easier said than done if ruminating has become a habit. And as with all habits, patience and practise of new behaviours are essential.

- Say to yourself, 'Stop ruminating!'
- Calm yourself by breathing, relaxation, meditation or exercise.
- Question the value of ruminating. What would my friends say to me if they knew I was ruminating?
- Am I looking at the whole picture? Does it really matter that much?
- What would I say about this in five years' time? Will it be that important?
- Do I apply the same rules or standards to myself as I do to other people?
- Have I got the facts right?
- Am I just tired and irritable?

Challenge yourself with these questions and statements.

- Maybe there's been a mistake or I've misunderstood?
- Have I checked that there is no other reason for this situation?
- Have I explained myself clearly?
- Maybe I jump to conclusions too quickly?
- I will act when I'm calm and have thought about it clearly.
- Ruminating like this is most likely harming me.

Mindfulness

When people dwell on anger or injustices they tend to revisit past situations or go into the future and fantasize about revenge. So bringing your mind into the present moment can be a powerful strategy. Say to yourself, 'Be here now!'

One mindfulness technique is to make a conscious effort at certain times of the day to focus your mind on your senses and become aware of everything that is around you: the sights, sounds, smells and textures.

Dealing with aggression online

In one of the cases reported in Chapter 1, a man made menacing online threats, including physical harm, against the MP Stella Creasy after she campaigned to put an image of Jane Austen on the new £10 note. The man used a number of Twitter accounts to retweet sinister posts and send a series of menacing messages directly to the MP. In another sad and tasteless online incident, a man left obscene messages and videos on a condolence page set up by the family of a 15-year-old girl who had committed suicide. He had never met the girl in question.

Anonymity is one aspect behind aggressive online behaviour and its main attraction to those who indulge in it. People are more aggressive and forthright online because they are anonymous and can act unpleasantly without immediate consequence. Operating undercover enables people do things they wouldn't ordinarily do. As mentioned in Chapter 1, psychologist John Suler identified six factors that could combine to change people's behaviour online: dissociative anonymity ('My actions can't be attributed to my person'); invisibility ('Nobody can tell what I look like, or judge my tone'); asynchronicity ('My actions do not occur in real time'); solipsistic introjection ('I can't see these people, I have to guess at who they are and their intent'); dissociative imagination ('This is not the real world and these are not real people'); and minimizing authority ('There are no authority figures here, so I can act freely').

The combination of any number of these leads to people behaving in ways they wouldn't when away from the screen and can lead to them abusing other people on the internet in ways they wouldn't dream of in real life. Recent research suggests people who engage in online trolling may have dark personalities and are examples of everyday sadists. Researchers conducted two online studies with over 1,200 people, giving personality tests to each subject along with a survey about their internet commenting behaviour.[1] They were looking for evidence that linked trolling with the 'dark tetrad' of personality traits: narcissism, sociopathy, Machiavellianism and sadism. They found that these antisocial personality traits were highest among people who said trolling was their favourite internet activity. The study found that trolls operate as agents of chaos, exploiting issues to make other users appear overly emotional or foolish in some manner. If an unfortunate person falls into their trap of responding defensively, the trolling intensifies, indicating that trolls feel sadistic pleasure at the distress of others. Individuals possessing sadistic personalities tend to display recurrent aggressive behaviour. This can include the use of emotional cruelty and purposefully manipulating others through the use of fear. Brain-scanning studies show that feeling pleasure at others' misfortune (sadism or *schadenfreude*, as it is sometimes termed) is associated with those individuals who experience high levels of envy and low self-esteem.[2]

Online harassment is on the increase and the problem of cyber-harassment has escalated in recent times. Some individuals on the receiving end, including those prominent in politics and the world of celebrity, have taken to naming and shaming and/or prosecuting those who are aggressive online.

Cyberbullying, e-bullying or trolling is intrusive and a form of psychological abuse. It takes place through smartphones and tablets using social networking sites, messaging apps, gaming sites and chat rooms such as Facebook, XBox Live, Instagram, YouTube and Snapchat. According to Bullying UK, an online resource, cyber-harassment is the act of sending offensive, rude and insulting messages and being abusive. It may involve behaviour such as that described below.

- **Denigration** This is when someone sends information about another person that is false, damaging and untrue, perhaps sharing photos of someone for the purpose of ridicule, spreading fake rumours and gossip.
- **Flaming** When someone is purposely using really extreme and offensive language and getting into online arguments and fights. People do this to cause reactions and enjoy the fact that it causes someone else to get distressed.
- **Impersonation** Someone will hack into a person's email or social networking account and use that person's online identity to send or post vicious or embarrassing material to and about others.
- **Outing and trickery** This is when someone may share personal information about another person or trick someone into revealing secrets and then forward them to others. They may do this with private images and videos, too. This can take the form of 'doxing' (sometimes written as 'doxxing' – see last entry in the list). The term derives from the abbreviation 'docs' (documents). It is an activity in which someone openly reveals and publicizes information about an individual for revenge via the violation of privacy.

- **Cyberstalking** The act of repeatedly sending messages that include threats of harm, harassment, intimidating messages or engaging in other online activities that make a person afraid for his or her safety.
- **Exclusion** When people intentionally leave someone out of a group, such as group messages, online apps, gaming sites and other online engagement. It is a form of social mistreatment.
- **Doxing or doxxing** This is a controversial issue that highlights the conflicts surrounding freedom of information. An internet-based group of 'hacktivists', Anonymous, became known for a series of high-profile publicity stunts, distributing denial-of-service attacks on government and corporate websites, making frequent use of doxing. Related groups are AntiSec and LulzSec, the latter coming to international prominence after hacking the websites of the Public Broadcasting Service, Sony and the United States Senate. These groups claim that they aim to protest government censorship and monitoring of the internet. Supporters call members of these groups 'freedom fighters' and digital Robin Hoods, while critics describe them as 'cyber lynch-mobs' or 'cyber terrorists'.

Curbing cyber-aggression

The general advice is to ignore rather than engage with online aggressors. It is not uncommon to use the phrase, 'Please do not feed the trolls', along with accompanying signs. This advice has, for several years, been suggested as the way to curb trolls online, but not everyone agrees ignoring them is the right thing to do. Some people argue that if 'feeding the trolls' provokes or encourages them in the short term, in the long term, sustained resistance and a confident attitude of intolerance to harassment is the only way to create the impression that something has to and can change.

If you post abuse about anyone online, or if you send threats, you can be traced by the police without any difficulty. Every visit you make to a website shows up as an electronic note of your activity. Even if you create an anonymous email address using Gmail, Hotmail or Yahoo, you can still be traced.

You can keep yourself safe from online aggressors by taking the steps listed next.

- Change your passwords regularly and use a combination of letters, lower and upper case, symbols and numbers. Don't use any part of your name or email address and don't use your birth date, because that will make it easy for people who know you to guess. Don't let anyone see you signing in; if they do, change your password as soon as you can.
- If you are using a public computer, such as in a library, computer shop or a shared family computer, be sure to sign out of any web service you are using before leaving the computer, so that you can protect your privacy.
- Never give your password to anyone.
- Don't provide your credit card number or other identifying information as proof of age to access or subscribe to a website run by any person or company you are not personally familiar with or that doesn't have an extremely good, widespread reputation.
- Think twice before you post anything online because, once it's out there, you can't take it back. It is easy for any comments or posts you make online to be taken out of context and these could be damaging to you in the long term.
- Block or ignore unwanted users.
- If a forum or chat room becomes stressful, leave it.
- Instruct children not to give out personal information online – real name, address or phone number – without your permission.
- Be very cautious about putting any pictures of yourself or your children online anywhere or allowing anyone else (schools, sports associations) to publish any photos. Some stalkers become obsessed because of an image.

How to deal with cyber-harassment

Stop contact

Advice from Working to Halt Online Abuse (WHOA), an organization that fights online harassment, states that as soon as you determine that you are being harassed by someone, tell that person in clear terms to stop contacting you and leave it there. You do not need to explain why; just state that you do not want the person to contact you.

Keep the message safely for your records. A first reaction when we are on the receiving end of harassment may well be to delete any harassing communications we have received, but it is important to save every communication you have had with the harasser. If you receive phone calls from the harasser, your local phone company can help you trace them. Do not destroy any evidence and, as soon as you can, give the evidence to the police.

Complain to the appropriate parties

It can at times be a little difficult for people to determine who the appropriate party is to complain to. If you're harassed in a chat room, contact whoever runs the server you were using. If you're harassed on any kind of instant messaging service, read the terms of service and harassment policies that are provided and use any contact address given there. If someone has created a website to harass you, complain to the server where the site is hosted. If you're being harassed via email, complain to the email service (such as Hotmail) used to send the messages.

Hold the harasser to account

If the circumstances and behaviour of the harasser are threatening to your safety and well-being, report the harasser to the police. However, online communication is near impossible to police effectively and doing so could have dire consequences for freedom of speech. Perhaps the best way of dealing with online negative and aggressive behaviour is for more of us to be persuaded not to engage in it and thus help make it socially unacceptable. Therefore, we each need to do our individual bit online to assert pro-social communication over antisocial forms and be unafraid of challenging those who engage in hostile lines of attack.

Laws

It is useful to know of UK legislation that covers online harassment. In the UK, contributions made to the internet are covered by the Malicious Communications Act 1988, as well as the Communications Act 2003. Under section 127 of the 2003 Act, jail sentences were limited to a maximum of six months. This Act was drawn up before the popularization of social networking and it could not have been foreseen how pervasive social networking would become. There remains ambiguity over what constitutes a public communications system. Twitter and Facebook are 'public' in the sense that they are free to use and open to view unless specified otherwise, but they are not public services; they are profit-making companies funded by investors and advertising.

Between 2003 and 2011 there were 5,316 people found guilty at magistrates' courts in England and Wales of offences under section 127. These figures include obscene telephone calls and text messages as well as internet-based communications. The Criminal Justice and Courts Act 2015 amended the earlier Act to introduce time limits where the offence may be tried within three years of the alleged offence and within six months of evidence coming to the knowledge of the prosecutor. Sending messages that are 'grossly offensive or of an indecent, obscene or menacing character' is an offence whether they are received by the intended recipient or not.

Some people have been imprisoned in the UK for online harassment. Frank Zimmerman, for example, was given a 26-week jail sentence, suspended for two years, after making email threats to the MP Louise Mensch; Joshua Cryer was given a two-year community order of 240 hours of community service for racist tweets directed at footballer Stan Collymore; Matthew Woods was sentenced to 12 weeks' imprisonment in a Young Offender Institution for posting offensive jokes about missing children April Jones and Madeleine McCann on Facebook.

In the next chapter, I discuss how to recover from relational and verbal forms of abuse and build emotional resilience to cope better with hostilities in daily life.

8

'Cruel words never hurt me'

The old truism, 'Cruel words never hurt me', turns out to be false. Many of us have grown up with this saying and see the connection between social and physical pain as only a figurative one, but it is not true: cruel words *do* hurt. Exposure to verbal abuse, even without physical abuse, has a strong effect on physical and psychological health. In this chapter, I highlight ways to build skills and the emotional wherewithal to withstand callous behaviour as we go about our daily lives.

An overlap between physical and social pain

Anyone can experience verbal abuse. People targeted by verbal abuse over time may succumb to a stress-related illness. Verbal abuse creates emotional pain and mental anguish in its target. As highlighted in earlier chapters, verbal abuse is the infliction of mental anguish and fear. Among other things, being verbally abused can involve being the target of someone else's abusive anger, or their accusations, or becoming a scapegoat. Verbal abuse can involve judging and criticizing someone, calling the person names, ordering them about or undermining them in some way; and it can be about discrimination on the grounds of differences including age, religion, race, gender and sexuality.

Exposure to verbal abuse has a negative effect on physical and psychological well-being, which is often unrecognized. Researchers have shown that verbal abuse in spousal and long-term relationships can have as great a psychological effect as physical abuse.[1] Furthermore, people exposed to long periods of verbal aggression may have difficulty forming conclusions and making decisions, feel that there is something wrong with them (selfish, too sensitive, crazy, for example), doubt their ability to communicate and experience self-doubt and low self-confidence.

Verbal abuse also heightens the chances of individuals experiencing anxiety and depression. At its most extreme, and after prolonged exposure to verbal abuse, individuals can experience clinical depression and post-traumatic stress disorder.

And the impact of verbal abuse is not just psychological; there are physical impacts on health too. Long-term effects of verbal aggression include physical symptoms such as chronic pain, migraine and frequent headaches, stammering, ulcers and gastrointestinal problems, as well as stress-related heart conditions. Furthermore, a rare but lethal heart condition caused by acute emotional distress known as 'stress cardiomyopathy' has been identified by scientists involved in neuroimaging studies, which show overlap in the brain regions involved in processing physical pain with those tied to social anguish.

The human brain and the way it responds to rewards and threats is shaped in early life. It is known that early childhood sexual abuse, physical abuse, or witnessing domestic violence, can cause abnormal physical changes in the brain of children. Furthermore, research suggests that not just physical abuse but also verbal abuse can leave a structural imprint on the developing brain. As mentioned in Chapter 1, studies by psychiatrist Dr Martin Teicher and colleagues from Harvard Medical School showed that individuals who reported experiencing verbal abuse from their peers during childhood and teenage years had underdeveloped connections between the left and right sides of their brain. The study revealed this same group of individuals had higher levels of anxiety, depression, anger, hostility, dissociation and drug abuse than others in the study.

Verbal abuse affects the brain because the teenage years are a period when brain connections are developing. The connection between abuse and the brain involves stress hormones. Harsh punishment, unwanted sexual advances, belittling and neglect are thought to release a cascade of chemicals, which produces an enduring effect on the signals that brain cells send and receive from each other. As a result, the brain becomes conditioned to over-respond to stress. If the findings of this study are to be believed, modern conditions or attitudes that tolerate verbal abuse put children at risk of developing brain abnormalities and elevate the risk of mental health problems.

In a review of studies on the connections between physical and social pain published in 2012, scientists offered an evolutionary explanation for the relationship.[2] They suggest that early humans needed social bonds to survive; acquiring food, eluding predators and nursing offspring are all easier done in partnership with others. This social alert system connected onto the physical pain system, so people could recognize social distress and quickly correct it. Some researchers even go so far as to suggest that feeling 'hurt' by being socially excluded may have been an adaptive way to prevent it.

One of the biggest hurdles to dealing with aggression is ourselves. Our survival apparatus is sometimes at odds with itself and we fight off threats and attacks with callousness, hostility, even violence. And so aggression and violence escalate in our culture. Dr Kathleen Taylor, author of a book entitled *Cruelty*, suggests there are mechanisms that drive us to behave in aggressive ways. Rewards for hostility to 'others' include curiosity, the desire for gain, competition for resources, wanting to impress superiors, the thrill of physical exertion and the excitement of risk-taking – all of which can be powerful drivers, especially when we are confronted with new and threatening situations. Threats, like rewards, are key to hostility and aggression. Humans have evolved threat responses associated with overpowering emotions designed to mobilize them to take action: fear for threats to existence, rage for threats to power, status or resources and disgust for intangible threats.

So, can we stop ourselves being aggressive? We could attempt to reduce the triggers for aggression and we could make individual and cultural changes to render aggression less socially acceptable. Aggression is a behaviour – something people know that they are doing – so aggression is something we can do less of if we so choose. There is potential for finding new ways of holding our own and asserting ourselves. If we learn to identify and describe our thoughts and emotions, we change them. We can build emotional resilience to help us find alternative means of coping with aggression and fear-making situations in daily life.

Emotional resilience

Knowing how to communicate clearly and with sensitivity can help you to avoid problems before they start. To be emotionally resilient means being able to spring back emotionally after suffering through difficult and stressful times in your life. Some people remain trapped in these negative emotions long after the stressful events that caused them have passed. Emotionally resilient people, however, are quickly able to bounce back to their normal emotional state. Emotional and physical resilience is, to a degree, something you are born with and some factors aren't under your control, such as age, gender and exposure to trauma, but it is possible for all of us to cultivate more of it. One key is adjusting how we think about adversity. Resilience refers to our capacity to deal with discomfort and adversity, and it is the same traits that make us more resilient that most often enrich our lives.

Resilient people view a difficulty as a challenge, not as something that they can't cope with. They look at their failures and mistakes as lessons to be learned from and opportunities for growth. They don't view them as a negative reflection on themselves. Resilient people don't paper over the negative emotions, but instead let them sit side by side with other feelings. So while they may be thinking, 'I'm scared about this', they are also likely to be thinking, 'but I know I can deal with it'. The resilient person also focuses on situations and events that they have control over; spending time worrying about uncontrollable events can often make us feel lost, helpless and powerless to take action.

Resilient people often rely on certain skills and competencies, as described below.

Assertiveness

Aggressive communication conveys a lack of respect for the other party. A better way to communicate involves assertiveness. Being assertive means communicating respect for yourself and for those you are communicating with. An assertive person communicates freely, but in a respectful, non-threatening manner. Assertiveness requires sensitivity for the feelings of other people and social awareness. It is a skill that can be learned and cultivated. One way to approach being more assertive is to assume that the person you're speaking with has no idea what it is you want from them. Ask for what you want explicitly and do so in a respectful tone of voice. Be prepared to say 'no'. It is OK to refuse any request or action that you believe is unreasonable. Also be prepared to follow through when you make promises, or say you will instigate a boundary to protect your personal space. Breaking promises or reneging on a boundary undermines the power of your words and lessens the trust others have in you.

Steps you can take away from anger and towards assertive communication include these.

1 **Pausing to interrupt your initial angry impulse** This way you can think up a more considered response.

2 **Taking time out** Don't respond until you are calm and have identified the things that triggered your anger.

3 **Communicating** Respond only when you are calm. Make it clear that you will defend yourself if necessary, but that you are not on the attack. Talk about how you have been affected by what has been said. Talk about your own experience to get your message across. Then seek the other person's cooperation to find a way forward that will work for you both.

Personal boundaries

To maintain an assertive stance in daily life we need personal boundaries. Personal boundaries are the imaginary lines we draw around ourselves to protect us from the behaviour or demands of other people. Usually at the root of personal boundary issues is fear – the fear that we aren't good enough or deserving as we are.

For many of us personal boundaries require us to adopt a new mindset. Having personal boundaries is perfectly acceptable. It doesn't mean that you are selfish or uncaring. It is both completely acceptable and absolutely necessary for healthy relationships. It may be that you have been allowing others to take advantage of you and you might have been put in situations that are really unacceptable to you. Defining your values, your belief system and your outlook on life can help you to get a clear picture of who you are and how you want to live.

Personal boundaries have a lot to do with self-efficacy. Self-efficacy reflects our confidence in our ability to exert control over our own motivation, behaviour and social environment. Unless you believe that your actions can produce the outcomes you desire, you will have little incentive to act or to persevere in the face of difficulties. This touches virtually every aspect of our lives: how we face adversity, our vulnerability to stress and depression and the decisions we make.

When you define and implement personal boundaries in your life, you will feel more empowered and self-confident and this will be conveyed in the way you communicate and conduct yourself in everyday life. Respecting boundaries goes both ways, however. Individually, we need also to examine our own behaviour and words to see where we might be crossing other people's boundaries. Then we can work to change those behaviours so that we are reflecting the respect and support we want for ourselves. Certain beliefs about ourselves or certain situations can make us fearful. When we are aware of aroused feelings, this is a signal to pause, take stock of our feelings and instigate personal boundaries.

Every emotionally charged situation includes three things:

- the activating event;
- the targeted person's beliefs about the activating event;
- the targeted person's resulting feelings or behaviours.

Too often, we jump straight to the feelings or behaviours about the event, without pausing to consider our beliefs. If we change our beliefs about the aggressive event, it can help us change our response to it.

'I don't believe that people should control others so I won't put up with this controlling behaviour from him, or anybody.'

Furthermore, addressing the offensive or aggressive behaviour empowers the targeted person and sets the boundary for next time. Here's a suggested approach for setting boundaries in a hostile situation.

1 **Inform** Clearly describe the problem.
2 **Define the unacceptable** Let the other person know what it is about his or her behaviour that is not acceptable.
3 **Share your emotions** Let the other person know how the situation made you feel.
4 **Request the solution you seek** Suggest to the other person the solution you seek.
5 **Let him or her know the alternatives** Let the other person know what you plan to do if he or she won't comply with your request.

Emotional awareness

Humans are highly capable and effective problem-solvers who can become stronger and more flexible in stressful times. Because of built-in survival mechanisms, our brains are naturally wired to pay more attention to negative events than positive ones, but one key to building resilience lies in noticing and appreciating positive experiences whenever and wherever they occur.

Emotionally resilient people are therefore emotionally aware people and likely to engage in mindful self-reflection. Even if you don't find that this comes naturally at first it is something that most of us can be become skilled at with practice. Pause for a few moments in your day to identify what you are feeling and why.

Emotionally resilient people look at the problem and say, 'What's the solution to that? What is this trying to teach me?' Looking at painful and difficult interactions as an opportunity to learn and problem-solve and building the confidence and the habit of moving towards the pain instead of running from it are ways of building resilience. When a problem arises, own what is happening to you. Use critical thinking, reasoning and problem-solving techniques on your own so you will trust your instincts more. Resist the urge to blame others. You are resourceful enough to find ways that work best for you.

Support

If you're lucky enough to have people around you to whom your existence matters, this can provide much-needed security. In fact, a study in the journal *Psychological Science* found that social support can relieve the intensity of physical pain.[3] The ease with which you are able to ask for and accept support from friends and family matters. If you can ask for help when others do not know that you need it, you may benefit from support that would not have otherwise been offered.

In addition to being around supportive people, being of service to others is a powerful way of strengthening resilience. In studies, researchers found that serotonin (the neurotransmitter associated with feelings of happiness and well-being) was used more efficiently by people who had just engaged in an act of kindness. Also, it is thought that receiving and appreciating kindness from others may be just as important as offering it to others, because gratitude is considered to be an important part of resilience. Learning to notice and to appreciate the positive things going on in your life is important. One way to do this is to consciously draw attention to the positive things and people in your life that you may have started taking for granted.

Keep a sense of humour

Laughing in the face of adversity can be profoundly pain-relieving, for both body and mind. Laughing reduces tension levels and psychologically can be empowering. Playing with a situation makes a person more powerful than sheer determination and more willing to muster the wherewithal and courage to assert themselves. A bit of gentle teasing or self-mockery can help. 'Hey, come on, Jane, stop being a scaredy-cat!'

Show empathy

One attribute that differentiates people with positive relationships from people who struggle to maintain relationships is the ability to be compassionate and empathetic. Empathy helps build our own self-worth and see ourselves and everyone around us as having value, yet not putting down or enabling anyone. To be compassionate means being aware of and responsive to the suffering of others. To be empathetic means being able to notice the verbal and non-verbal signals people give out that alert you to what they need or want. People who do not have the ability to recognize these cues are at a great social disadvantage in terms of the way they communicate with others.

Empathy is perhaps the single most powerful communication skill you can learn to use in everyday situations to counter aggression. Empathy involves an openness to engage emotionally with the other person. Though you are not able to feel exactly what another person is feeling – nor do you try – making use of your abilities to empathize can allow you to consider how the other person feels and helps you to see that someone else's perspective is either similar to or different from your own. This gives us the opportunity to resolve conflicts when they arise that take account of and are respectful of differences in points of view.

These abilities and competencies can help you cope well in stressful situations and help you 'in the moment' during aggressive encounters. The next and final chapter looks at what it takes to build empathy and how individually we can do our bit to lessen aggression in everyday life.

9

The way forward – building a language of empathy

> When a child hits a child, we call it aggression.
> When a child hits an adult, we call it hostility.
> When an adult hits an adult, we call it assault.
> When an adult hits a child, we call it discipline.
>
> Haim G. Ginott (psychotherapist, 1922–73)

Aggression is usually directed towards people and most people who are targets of aggression get angry in return. So how do we avoid tit-for-tat behaviour and lessen aggression in daily life? In this final chapter, a way forward is suggested – the encouragement of empathic expression in everyday life, something that requires the adoption and spread of a language of its own.

A lot of us may show aggression when we are fearful. Acknowledging fear, recognizing when we feel scared and admitting it, if only to ourselves, may help us feel a sense of compassion for ourselves, which is the starting point for helping ourselves.

We often have a tendency to blame others for doing or saying things that scare us, but if we take back the responsibility for our feelings, we can change the emotional state we are in. Expressing, or at least recognizing, the fear that we feel can help to get us out of a stuck place and mobilize us into action. In other words, when we acknowledge our fears, this usually has the effect of dissipating them.

So being cognizant of your feelings helps. And be prepared to take risks as well. Be willing to be bold and courageous, even if you feel scared. Learn to walk with fear as if it's your travelling companion, even if it is uninvited company. It does not have to block your way. Just acknowledge that it is there. Your legs may shake and your voice might quiver, but take a risk, make a request, try something new to allow yourself to move through your fear. What we need to keep fear in check and to stop it overwhelming us is a way of asserting ourselves that doesn't worsen the threat of violence and aggression.

Building a language of empathy in culture

Confronting fearful feelings in ourselves is only part of the solution. Our mode of expression and our language – body language and verbal language – make a lot of difference too. Language shapes our ideas and perceptions and, ultimately, our behaviour and actions. So if language plays a major role in shaping our social reality, then humans should be able to alter the way they communicate with each other to construct a non-violent social world. Language influences social norms in the sense that speaking is action intended to accomplish a specific purpose.

There are four aspects of interpersonal communication. First, there is the encoding/decoding aspect, where words are used to convey meaning. Second is the intention of the communication, where we establish whether the words used are meant to be taken literally or non-literally. Third is the perspective-taking aspect, where messages become vehicles that convey the speaker's intentions, but since the recipients may hold a different perspective, the same message can convey different meanings to them. Last, there is the dialogue itself, which is a joint activity. It can end up a cooperative activity where two people work together, or it can end up in misinterpretation, hostility and conflict.

Empathic language, which most likely developed to assist humans in creating a sense of communality, has the potential to provide a way forward. Empathy plays a large part in the act of cooperation. We need to pay close attention to the activities and goals of others to cooperate effectively. Furthermore, feelings and emotions generally win over rules. We rely more on what we *feel* than what we *think* when solving moral dilemmas.

Showing empathy does not mean that we agree with the other person and it does not mean that we have to accept what they are saying. It simply entails acknowledging the issue and any attendant frustration that goes with it, in order to suggest a reasonable way to deal with the situation. As the renowned psychologist Carl Rogers (1902–87) once said, 'Real communication occurs when we listen with understanding – to see the idea and attitude from the other person's point of view, to sense how it feels to them, to achieve their frame of reference in regard to the thing they are talking about.'

Empathic language demonstrates to the other person that you are concerned about them and have the ability to 'feel what they feel'. Empathy is an important social skill; empathically attuned people are generally cooperative sorts who are able to form healthy relationships. Empathy leads to a reciprocal liking of you and hence increases the other person's trust and relationship with you.

Some people are more empathic than others and the language people use reveals a lot about their levels of empathy. As illustrated in Chapter 2 (see Table 1, p. 21), there is a whole spectrum of what could be described as potential deficits or lack of empathy, but most of us can improve our empathy if we keep our moral–emotional apparatus in good working order. The good news is that empathy is contagious. The behaviours of people who display caring and trusting non-verbal behaviours, such as nods of the head, smiles and eye contact, while listening to other people, are quickly noticed by others and their behaviour has a positive influence on the rest of us.

The more people who express empathic concern for one another, the more others around them are likely to do their bit as well. American researchers Nicholas Christakis and James Fowler suggest that we are influenced by the moods of friends. Their experiments revealed that social networks have significant influence on individuals' behaviour. And surprisingly, the social influence does not end with those people we know and have some connection with. We influence our friends, who in their turn influence their friends, meaning that our actions can influence people we have never met.[1] In their book *Connected,* Christakis and Fowler claim that society should use the knowledge about social networks and the power and influence of social diffusion in order to create a better society.[2]

It may not be that we need to fix people who exhibit negative social traits, but we should recognize they may need more understanding and encouragement to adopt these social skills. Emotional self-management, practising interpersonal skills and social problem-solving are ways in which we can learn to show more empathy and reduce fear and aggression. These approaches provide a means of helping individuals moderate surging angry moods and may prevent individuals having to deal with another difficult emotion – guilt.

The ability to understand that different people have different points of view is a very healthy one. An inability to do this can bring judgement and attract conflict. So, in an argument, if we try not to hurt the other person's feelings and try to imagine how they must be feeling (empathy), it will stop us expressing hostility or exacerbating aggression. Blaming the other person and viewing it as their problem is non-empathy. Empathy goes hand in hand with social skills and a lack of it goes hand in hand antisocial skills. Empathic language provides us with ways to soothe the emotional state of another and mobilize ourselves and other people into action.

Here are some tips for maintaining respectful communication when interacting with other people.

- **Listen well** When stressed, we tend to listen less well; try to relax and listen carefully to the views and feelings of others. Ask for clarification and reflect back what you thought was said to demonstrate that you are trying to comprehend the other person's perspective.
- **Know your boundaries** Know what you will tolerate and not tolerate in terms of behaviour from others. Put in place a behavioural line that cannot be crossed. Your enforcement of these boundaries is the primary way to protect yourself.
- **Be alert to what others say and don't say, what they do and don't do** Ignore comments such as, 'Nobody else minds, so why should I?' or people who tell you to 'Lighten up' or say, 'Who cares anyway?' Act on matters that you are impassioned about and concern you.
- **Learn to tolerate challenging experiences** Pain is painful, stress is stressful, fear is inevitable at times. Resilient people understand that stress, fear and anger are part of everyday experience. It is better to come to terms with these experiences and feelings. It is better to learn to experience the full range of emotions, trusting that we will bounce back.
- **Mind your language** Words have power and our responses can either exacerbate aggression or help reduce it. Using the language of empathy, that recognizes the value of the other person

and acknowledges his or her perspective, will help to diminish aggression. When imposing boundaries, an approach that is 'fair but firm' is what we need to aim for.

- **Challenge your own prejudices** Take time to analyse your own prejudices, biases and assumptions about others. When we are prejudiced, we violate three standards: reason, justice and tolerance.

- **Remember that well-managed conflict can be constructive** especially if those involved use it as an opportunity to increase understanding and find a way forward together out of the conflict situation.

- **Trust people and treat them with respect** Try to treat other people as if they are just as important as you. Trusting (but not naive) people tend to be happier, better liked by others, more honest and more moralistic than less trusting people. Conversely, distrust puts up barriers to relationships.

- **Be self-compassionate** Showing yourself small kindnesses each day should help you to express empathy for others more readily.

- **Be an active helper** Helping others can make you healthier, happier and less stressed because it releases endorphins to produce a 'rush' that is referred to as the 'helper's high'. Studies have shown that helping others can produce feelings of happiness and activate reward centres in the brain in the same way as can food or drugs.

Beyond skilling ourselves up, the big challenge for us all, as the internet age advances, is working out how social networking technology can harness the power of empathy to enhance social interaction. Social media such as Twitter may inspire people to social action, but empathic connection will only happen if social networks learn to spread it. It matters what language we use in our daily interactions; as stated previously, language shapes our ideas and perceptions and plays a major role in shaping our social reality.

The writer Margaret J. Wheatley once remarked, 'Aggression only moves in one direction – it creates more aggression.' From observation and experience this seems to ring true. Empathy, however, shows that we acknowledge and show sensitive regard for the feelings of others and in so doing we transform the way in which we resolve conflicts. Not only can exercising our empathy make us more empathic in daily life, it makes us happier people because it helps life feel more meaningful. Our own problems drift to the periphery of the mind and seem smaller, and we increase our capacity for connection or compassionate action.

Empathy comes through becoming self-aware and having a clear perception of your own personality – your thoughts, beliefs, motivations and emotions. Self-awareness allows you to understand yourself and, by doing so, understand other people and your responses to them. Hence empathetic people are able to make friends and keep them, because they can see things from another person's point of view.

Showing our empathy for other people has physical benefits, too, for it fosters deep social connections and people with a strong support network tend to live longer. For above all, empathy is a reciprocal asset. What enables people to get along with each other is each person's ability to empathize with the other. When we place ourselves in others' shoes and feel what they are feeling we not only mirror the distress of the other people, but are moved to respond in helping ways. In other words, empathy helps us take care of one another. It is mutual aid.

In the end, however, whether or not we make the most of empathy – the glue that keeps us sticking together and cooperating – rests with each of us doing our bit to make the world of human interaction a better, less hostile place. So it is up to each and every one of us to understand and regulate ourselves and our emotions so that we can get along with others. In order to do this, we need a language of empathy to bring radical change and benefit to human relationships. The change begins when we accept that a new way is needed and we enthusiastically opt in and start communicating afresh.

Useful addresses

Bullying UK
Website: www.bullying.co.uk/
cyberbullying
Helpline: 0808 800 2222

Galop
Website: www.galop.org.uk
Helpline: 0800 999 5428
Offers support for lesbian, gay,
bisexual and transgender (LGBT)
people experiencing domestic
violence.

National Stalking Helpline
Website: www.suzylamplugh.
org/Pages/Category/
national-stalking-helpline
Helpline: 0808 802 0300

Refuge
Website: www.refuge.org.uk
Helpline: 0808 2000 247

Respect
Website: www.respectphoneline.
org.uk
Helpline: 0808 802 4040
Support services and programmes
for men and women who inflict
violence in relationships. They also
provide an advice line for men who
are victims of domestic violence.

Victim Support
Website: www.victimsupport.org.uk
Helpline: 0808 1689 111
Offers free and confidential help
to victims of crime, their families,
friends and anyone else affected.

Women's Aid
Website: www.womensaid.org.uk
Helpline: 0808 2000 247

**Working to Halt Online Abuse
(WHOA)**
Website: www.haltabuse.org

Notes

Introduction

1 Galen, C. (1963) *On the Passions and Errors of the Soul* (trans. P. W. Harkins). Columbus, OH: Ohio University Press (original work written *c*.AD 180). P. 38.
2 Aristotle (1931) *The Works of Aristotle* (ed. W. D. Ross). Oxford: Clarendon Press (original work written *c*.350 BC).
3 Aquinas, T. (1964) *Summa Theologiae* (Compendium of Theology). London: Blackfriars (original work completed *c*.1273).
4 Averill, J. R. (1982) *Anger and Aggression: An essay on emotion*. New York: Springer-Verlag.
5 Scherer, K. R., Wallbott, H. G. and Summerfield, A. B. (1986) *Experiencing Emotion: A cross-cultural study*. Cambridge: Cambridge University Press.
6 Lazarus, R. S. (1991) *Emotion and Adaption*. Oxford: Oxford University Press.
7 Bègue, L., Beauvois, J.-L., Courbet, D., Oberlé, D., Lepage, J. and Duke, A. A. (2015) 'Personality predicts obedience in a Milgram paradigm', *Journal of Personality*, 83(3): 299–306.
8 Baas, M., De Dreu, C. K. W. and Nijstad, B. A. (2011) 'Creative production by angry people peaks early on, decreases over time, and is relatively unstructured', *Journal of Experimental Social Psychology*, 47 (6): 1107–15.
9 Aarts, H., Ruys, K. I., Veling, H., Renes, R. A., de Groot, J. H. B., van Nunen, A. M. and Geertjes, S. (2010) 'The art of anger: reward context turns avoidance responses to anger-related objects into approach', *Psychological Science*, 21(10): 1406–10.
10 Kring, A. M. (2000) 'Gender and anger', in A. H. Fischer (ed.), *Gender and Emotion: Social psychological perspectives*. Cambridge: Cambridge University Press. Pp. 211–231.
11 Evers, C., Fischer, A. H., Rodriguez Mosquera, P. M. and Manstead, A. S. R. (2005) 'Anger and social appraisal: A "spicy" sex difference?', *Emotion*, 5(3): 258–66.
12 Thomas, S. P. (1993) *Women and Anger*. New York: Springer.
13 DiGiuseppe, R. and Tafrate, R. C. (2004) *The Anger Disorder Scale Manual*. Toronto: Multi-Health Systems.

1 Recognizing aggression

1 Thomas, S. P. (2003) 'Anger: The mismanaged emotion', *Dermatology Nursing*, 15(4): 351–7. See also S. P. Thomas, C. Smucker and P. Droppleman (1998) 'It hurts most around the heart: A phenomenolog-

ical exploration of women's anger', *Journal of Advanced Nursing*, 28(2): 311–22.

2 Teicher, M. H., Samson, J. A., Polcari, A. and McGreenery, C. E. (2006) 'Sticks, stones and hurtful words: Relative effects of various forms of childhood maltreatment', *American Journal of Psychiatry*, 163: 993–1000. Also J. Choi, B. Jeong, M. L. Rohan, A. M. Polcari and M. H. Teicher (2009) 'Preliminary evidence for white matter tract abnormalities in young adults exposed to parental verbal abuse', *Biological Psychiatry*, 65(3): 227–34.

3 Suler, J. (2004) 'The online disinhibition effect', *Cyberpsychology and Behaviour*, 7(3): 321–6.

4 Buckels, E. E., Trapnell, P. D. and Paulhus, D. L. (2014) 'Trolls just want to have fun', *Personality and Individual Differences*, 67: 97–102.

5 An article on the case can be found on the BBC's website at: <www.bbc.co.uk/news/uk-england-berkshire-14897948>.

2 Common lines of attack

1 Bianchi, E. C. (2014) 'Entering adulthood in a recession tempers later narcissism', *Psychological Science*, 25(7):1429–37.

2 S. Baron-Cohen (2011) *Zero Degrees of Empathy: A new theory of human cruelty*. London: Penguin.

3 Buckels, E. E., Jones, D. N. and Paulhus, D. L. (2013) 'Behavioral confirmation of everyday sadism', *Psychological Science*, 24(11): 2201–9.

4 Furham, A., Richards, S. C. and Paulhus, D. L. (2013) 'The dark triad of personality: A 10-year review', *Social and Personality Psychology Compass*, 7(3): 199–216.

5 Harris, J. (2000) 'Home Office Research Study 203: An evaluation of the use and effectiveness of the Protection from Harassment Act 1997'. London: Research, Development and Statistics Directorate, Home Office.

6 Sheridan, L., Davies, G. and Boon, J. (2001) 'The course and nature of stalking: A victim perspective', *Howard Journal of Criminal Justice*, 40(3): 215–34.

7 Simon, G. (2010) *In Sheep's Clothing: Understanding and dealing with manipulative people*. Little Rock, AR: Parkhurst.

8 Zimmerman, A. G. (2012) 'Online Aggression: The influences of anonymity and social modelling'. Unpublished thesis, University of North Florida.

9 Hardaker, C. (2013) '"Uh . . . not to be nitpicky . . . but . . . the past tense of drag is dragged, not drug": An overview of trolling strategies', *Journal of Language Aggression and Conflict*, 1(1): 57–86.

3 Dealing with aggression without being aggressive

1 de Waal, F. (2010) *The Age of Empathy: Nature's lessons for a kinder society*. Toronto: McClelland and Stewart.

2 Mayer, J. D. and Salovey, P. (1997) 'What is emotional intelligence?', in P. Salovey and D. J. Sluyter (eds), *Emotional Development and Emotional Intelligence*. New York: Basic Books.

3 Miller, W. R. and Rollnick, S. (2013) *Motivational Interviewing: Helping people change* (third edition). New York: Guilford Press.

4 Hollander, M. (2015) 'The repertoire of resistance: Non-compliance with directives in Milgram's "obedience" experiments', *British Journal of Social Psychology*, 54(3): 425–44.

6 Bringing covert aggression into the open

1 Tsetsos, K., Chater, N. and Usher, M. (2012) 'Salience driven value integration explains decision biases and preference reversal', *Proceedings of the National Academy of Sciences*, 109(24): 9659–64.

7 Dealing with overt aggression

1 Buckels, E. E., Trapnell, P. D. and Paulhus, D. L. (2014) 'Trolls just want to have fun', *Personality and Individual Differences*, 67: 97–102.

2 Takahashi, H., Kato, M., Matsuura, M., Mobbs, D., Suhara, T. and Okubo, Y. (2009) 'When your gain is my pain and your pain is my gain: Neural correlates of envy and schadenfreude', *Science*, 323(5916): 937–9.

8 'Cruel words never hurt me'

1 O'Leary, K. D. (1999) 'Psychological abuse: A variable deserving critical attention in domestic violence', *Violence and Victims*, 14(1): 3–23.

2 Eisenberger, N. I. (2012) 'Broken hearts and broken bones: A neural perspective on the similarities between social and physical pain', *Current Directions in Psychological Science*, 21: 42–7.

3 Master, S. L., Eisenberger, N. I., Taylor, S. E., Naliboff, B. D., Shirinyan, D. and Lieberman, M. D. (2009) 'A picture's worth: Partner photographs reduce experimentally induced pain', *Psychological Science*, 20: 1316–18.

9 The way forward – building a language of empathy

1 Christakis, N. A. and Fowler, J. H. (2013) 'Social contagion theory: Examining dynamic social networks and human behavior', *Statistics in Medicine*, 32: 556–77.

2 Christakis, N. A. and Fowler, J. H. (2009) *Connected: The surprising power of our social networks and how they shape our lives – how your friends' friends' friends affect everything you feel, think, and do*. New York: Little Brown.

Index